THE ANTI-ANXIETY PROGRAM

Also Available

THE
anti-
anxiety
PROGRAM

a workbook of proven strategies
to overcome worry, panic, and phobias

SECOND EDITION

Peter J. Norton

Martin M. Antony

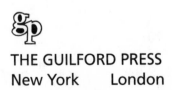

THE GUILFORD PRESS
New York   London

Copyright © 2021 The Guilford Press
A Division of Guilford Publications, Inc.
370 Seventh Avenue, Suite 1200, New York, NY 10001
www.guilford.com

See page 246 for terms of use for audio files.

Printed in the United States of America

Last digit is print number: 9   8   7   6   5   4   3   2   1

Library of Congress Cataloging-in-Publication Data is available from the publisher.

ISBN 978-1-4625-4361-8 (paperback) — ISBN 978-1-4625-4489-9 (hardcover)

To all of my patients, mentors, and students over the years—I have learned more from each of you than you could ever know. Thank you.

—P. J. N.

For my daughters, Sita and Kalinda.

—M. M. A.

acknowledgments

We would like to thank our editors at The Guilford Press, Kitty Moore and Christine Benton, for their guidance and encouragement throughout the process. A special acknowledgment to Professor Timothy Jones, DMA, who narrated the relaxation exercises that are available via the Guilford Press website, and Reynaldo Ochoa, DMA, who conducted the audio recording. At the time of the recording, both were on the faculty of the University of Houston Moores School of Music.

Finally, a thank-you to those who first developed, shaped, and studied many of the strategies described in this book, as well as to our mentors, who first exposed us to these approaches: David H. Barlow, Aaron T. Beck, Thomas Borkovec, Timothy A. Brown, David M. Clark, Michelle G. Craske, Edna B. Foa, Steven Hayes, Richard G. Heimberg, Debra Hope, Isaac Marks, Ron Norton, Lars-Goran Öst, Randy Paterson, S. Rachman, Ron Rapee, Paul Salkovskis, Richard Swinson, Maureen Whittal, Joseph Wolpe, and many others.

authors' note

All the individuals described in this workbook are heavily disguised composites of real people we have worked with and are intended to illustrate experiences we have observed often in our practices.

In this book, we alternate between masculine and feminine pronouns when referring to a single individual. We have made this choice to promote ease of reading as our language continues to evolve and not out of disrespect toward readers who identify with other personal pronouns. We sincerely hope that all will feel included.

contents

introduction
the faces of anxiety

Valerie paces around her apartment as she waits for her husband to arrive home from work. It's 6:00 P.M., and she wonders where he is. She tried calling him on his cell phone, but there was no answer. He normally finishes work at 5:00 P.M., and it only takes him about a half hour to get home. Her mind starts to race. What's making him late? Perhaps he's been in a terrible accident, she thinks. Maybe he's gotten fired and is drinking himself into a stupor at some bar. Could it be an affair? Valerie feels her emotions swing from worry to anger to terror. She's frustrated because there's nothing she can do but wait, so she pours herself another gin and tonic. Lately, she is starting to worry about how much she drinks. Her husband, Carl, has also commented that he is concerned about how much she is drinking, but Valerie feels that it's about the only thing that will take the edge off her emotions. About a half hour later, Carl walks in the door, explaining that there'd been construction on the highway and the traffic was backed up. Why hadn't he answered his cell phone? Simple: he didn't have it with him. Indeed, Valerie now notices it lying on an end table. She breathes a sigh of relief. Valerie had let her anxiety get the best of her. That had been happening a lot lately.

Jacob worries about his health. When he was a teenager, his father was complaining of a headache, then suddenly collapsed from a stroke and died in the hospital. While Jacob was at the hospital with his father, he saw many other stroke patients, some of whom couldn't speak, were partially paralyzed, or seemed like "vegetables." Ever since then, Jacob has been terrified of having a stroke or some other sudden major health problem. Whenever Jacob experiences a sharp headache, he immediately fears that he's having a stroke or an aneurysm. Terrified that he will die, Jacob rushes to the emergency room. Each time, the doctors run some tests and assure him that he isn't dying, and then he feels lucky, as though he has cheated death. But each time he also worries that the next time might really be a stroke. What's more, Jacob has started to worry about other health problems and is starting to have panic attacks. When he notices his heart rate speed up, he's convinced that he's having a heart attack. He avoids doing anything that might make his heart rate increase, like exercising or running, but he fears this is bad for his health and could increase his chances of developing a serious medical problem.

Bindi moved to the city to attend college 2 years ago but feels like a fish out of water. She had always been somewhat shy growing up in her rural community, but this is different. She had some friends back home, but she doesn't have any friends in the city or at the university. She rarely leaves her apartment unless she has to go to class or get groceries. She feels like she can't fit in, that people will judge her. She doesn't feel like she knows how to be cosmopolitan, to dress like everyone does here, to effortlessly glide into parties and gatherings. She has also never been so far from her people's traditional tribal lands for this long and worries that people in the city are judging her on her heritage and appearance. So she keeps to herself most of the time. Bindi longs to return home to her community but feels like she would be a disappointment to her family and community if she gave up on her education. She has been feeling hopeless and depressed for the past few months and has recently begun to have occasional thoughts that life "just isn't worth it." She doesn't want to take her own life, but she doesn't know who to talk to for help.

Jacqui is a new mom. Although she has never had significant problems with anxiety in the past, she now finds she has intrusive thoughts about harming her newborn daughter. For example, when changing her baby's diaper, she sometimes experiences thoughts of strangling or sexually abusing her daughter. The thoughts shock and scare her. She has no desire to do these things and would never act on the thoughts, but she worries that they're a sign that she might do something bad to her daughter or that she's a terrible mother. Jacqui knows such thoughts aren't normal, and she does everything she can to avoid thinking them. She tries not to be alone with her baby or to be around anything that could be used to hurt her baby (for example, knives). But the more she tries not to think about hurting her baby, the more upset she becomes when experiencing intrusive thoughts.

What do Valerie, Jacob, Bindi, and Jacqui have in common? Each of them experiences excessive or exaggerated anxiety and fear. Valerie never even considers many common possibilities for her husband's delay. Bindi's fear of socializing persists even though she has made friends with people before. Jacqui is terrified of her own thoughts, even though she knows she would never act on them. Jacob is convinced that his physical sensations are signs of an impending stroke, even though he generally is in good health. For Valerie, her anxiety is starting to lead to her drinking more than she thinks is wise. Bindi's anxiety has led to feelings of depression and some thoughts of suicide. Jacob's worries about his health have started causing him to have panic attacks.

These are the faces of anxiety. Sometimes it's easy to understand how anxiety begins, as with Jacob, whose anxiety developed after watching his father die from a stroke. Other times the anxiety may seem absurd or difficult to understand, like Jacqui's thoughts about harming her infant. Everyone experiences anxiety and fear from time to time, but for some of us the anxiety and fear take control. These emotions dictate what we can and can't do. These emotions fire us up, even when everyone else around us would say there's no cause for concern.

If you identify with Valerie, Jacob, Bindi, or Jacqui—or with some aspects of more than one of them—this book can help you take control of your life back from anxiety and fear. This is a workbook, which means we'll lead you through a series of proven steps and give you hands-on exercises for making progress toward easing anxiety little by little.

Is This Program for You?

You can use this book if:

- You experience frequent anxiety about things that don't seem to bother other people as much.

- You experience panic attacks.

- Your mind is frequently consumed by worries or traumatic memories that you can't get rid of.

- Your anxiety, fears, or worries keep you from being able to do the things or live the life that you want.

You may have been diagnosed with an anxiety disorder already, but that isn't necessary to benefit from this program. Quite a few people who experience problems with anxiety have never talked to a doctor or mental health professional and have never received a diagnosis. In Chapter 1, we'll tell you about some of the more common ways that people experience anxiety and how it can affect their lives.

We have tried to write this book in a way that most people will be able to understand, including teens and adults. Some of the sections might be a little difficult for children to understand, so if you are considering getting a book for a child, we would recommend finding one written specifically for children or for parents of children. Just flip to the Resources section at the back of the book for recommendations before you put this book back on the bookshelf.

You may have already tried different methods for overcoming your anxiety, including other self-help programs, therapy, or medication. You may be in therapy or on medications right now. These are all fine. Many people choose to use this book in their therapy sessions, and this program can be used if people currently take medication. We briefly discuss some of the more commonly prescribed medications in Chapter 1, although for most people who are not currently on medication, we usually recommend that you try the program first and then consider additional treatment (for example, psychotherapy and/or medication) if you feel like you need more help. Regardless, feel free to discuss your options with your physician to make sure you get the best advice for your situation.

Updates for the Second Edition

In this second edition of *The Anti-Anxiety Program,* we have updated both the information and the program to fit with the latest research and developments in cognitive-behavioral therapy, or CBT. Some of the most noteworthy updates include:

- An expanded set of chapters (Chapters 5, 6, and 7) focusing on identifying and challenging the thoughts, beliefs, and assumptions underlying your anxiety

- A new chapter (Chapter 13) on using mindfulness-based techniques to help with stress and anxiety

- Sections throughout the book designed to help keep your motivation strong throughout the program

- An easier set of recommendations and instructions for helping you decide which sections of the program will be most useful in helping you overcome your anxiety

- And finally, we follow the stories of the four people introduced on pages 1 and 2—Valerie, Jacob, Bindi, and Jacqui—in every chapter as they progress through the program.

In this edition you'll learn the most widely studied and accepted techniques that mental health professionals use to help people overcome problems of extreme anxiety. The chapters are organized to simulate the steps that an experienced therapist would take you through. Part I is "The Prep." First, we'll teach you what anxiety is and why yours has grown out of control. Then we'll guide you through a self-assessment to openly and honestly take stock of how anxiety affects you and your life. Although this workbook is for a wide audience of anxiety sufferers, it's carefully designed to help readers develop a self-help treatment plan designed specifically for them. The third chapter will involve some activities to help you build your motivation and commitment to reducing your anxiety and making positive changes in your life. In Chapter 4, we will show you how to use the results of your self-assessments to plan your own path through the program, tailoring the techniques presented in this book to your particular fears and worries.

Chapters 5 through 11 ("The Core Program") present the core strategies, which are based on CBT, by far the most widely accepted, studied, and proven psychological treatment for helping people overcome their fears. You will start by learning to identify the thoughts and assumptions that drive your fears and to practice techniques that will allow you to shift your anxiety-provoking thoughts to a more realistic place. With these skills, you will then begin to confront the situations, sensations, and intrusive thoughts that trigger your fear and anxiety. Don't be afraid! This will be a gradual process conducted at a manageable pace. Just work through the beginning sections of the book and practice the skills we recommend, and you'll be ready to confront the triggers that give rise to your anxieties.

In Part III (Additional Strategies), you will learn about other techniques that have been found to be useful, including techniques to help you relax and control the physical manifestations of your anxiety and techniques for dealing with situations more mindfully. In the last chapter of this book, "Conclusion: Living without Anxiety," we offer ways to help cement the changes you've made while working through this program: strategies for preventing your anxiety from returning, techniques for overcoming barriers that occasionally get in the way of recovery, and personal changes you can make for an anxiety-free lifestyle. Finally, at the end of the book, you'll find a Resources section that lists dozens of sources of information and help, including other books, mobile apps, online resources and videos, and mental health organizations that can help put you in contact with cognitive-behavioral therapists in your area.

You will need to fill out some of the forms in this workbook more than once. Where that is the case, we invite you to photocopy them or download and print extra copies (see the end of the Contents for information on doing so).

Is Self-Help Effective for Anxiety?

As you read through this book, you may wonder whether anxiety can be treated through self-help. The effectiveness of self-help programs such as this one is well documented. In 2012, a team of researchers—Catrin Lewis, Jennifer Pearce, and Jonathan Bisson—reviewed more than 30 studies in which people with anxiety disorders were treated using self-help programs. These studies together involved over 1,100 people with a range of anxiety problems. What they found when combining the results of the individual studies is that, on average, people with anxiety who worked through programs like this improved substantially compared to people who didn't. What's even more impressive is that another large study like the previous one, conducted in 2018 by Professor Gavin Andrews and his research team, found that CBT programs like this one were as effective when completed using self-help books or computerized self-help programs delivered over the Internet as when done face to face with a therapist.

Now, before we go ahead and get rid of all of the therapists in the world, studies like these don't tell us all of the details. First, most of the self-help programs reviewed in this study involved some degree of therapist support, such as periodic phone calls. It's also quite possible that self-help, whether using a book or the Internet, is effective for most people with more mild or moderate anxiety problems, but including a therapist is better when the anxiety problems are more severe. It also seems reasonable to guess that a therapist might be preferable for people who have difficulty sticking with treatment on their own. On the other hand, self-help may be an excellent option for people with anxiety problems who either don't have CBT therapists near them or can't afford therapy.

Recommendations for Working through This Program

Feel free to use this book in whatever way you think will be most helpful to you, but we do have some tips for how to get the most out of this self-help program:

1. Start by skimming the entire book, before doing any of the exercises, learning the skills, or practicing the techniques we offer. We want you to be familiar not only with the ideas and skills each chapter presents but also with the program as a whole. This program is designed to build upon the techniques you have learned and advances you have made in earlier sections, so it's important for you to see the "big picture" as you practice using particular strategies.

2. Next, work through the first four chapters ("The Prep") one at a time. They are designed to help you understand your anxiety more deeply and to develop a personalized plan for which of the techniques in the following chapters will be best for you to emphasize. In each of those chapters, there will be specific instructions for what to work on and signposts for when you're ready to move on. After you are ready, move on to the core program in Chapters 5–11 based on your personalized plan. Again, each chapter will give you clear instructions for when to move on. In Chapters 12 and 13, you will have an opportunity to try out additional strategies that you

may find helpful, and then in the Conclusion you will work through some steps to help make sure you maintain the gains you made in the program in the long run.

3. Use the troubleshooting sections that appear throughout the book for help with problems that sometimes arise for those working through the program. When you feel that something isn't working, these tips will give you suggestions for overcoming obstacles like these:

- Difficulty finding the time to stick to the program (for example, to complete homework practices)

- Coping with other psychological problems, such as depression or substance abuse

- Difficulty getting or staying motivated

- Life stress (at work, in relationships, or in other areas)

- Medical complications

- Lack of relevant skills (for example, communication skills, driving skills)

4. Make a commitment to immerse yourself fully in the steps outlined in this program for letting go of your anxiety, fear, phobias, obsessions, and compulsions. These techniques work! That's been demonstrated time and time again by scientists in controlled studies, by therapists in their work with clients, and by people just like you. But it doesn't happen by looking at words on a page. It will only happen by taking the ideas and recommendations on these pages and putting them into action in your life.

The four people we introduced you to earlier in this Introduction all committed themselves to overcoming their anxiety using this program. Throughout the book we will show you how Valerie, Jacob, Bindi, and Jacqui applied the skills and techniques to their own anxieties and fears. But here's a sneak preview of how each of them is doing today:

Looking back to how she was before, Valerie can't believe how exhausting life was when she was always worrying about meaningless little things. "It was like my brain was running a marathon every day!" she said. Since working through the program she finds that she can quickly shut down the worries if they get going, but more often than not, the worries and anxieties don't get started in the first place. In fact, she recounted taking a business trip out of town recently and forgetting to pack her phone charger. When her phone's battery died on the first day, she shrugged and reassured herself that everything would be fine at home even if she couldn't check in with Carl. She just picked up a new charger from a store the next morning before her meetings, and everything was fine. Valerie was also able to cut back on her drinking, since she didn't need to use alcohol to control her anxieties anymore.

Jacob made steady progress, though a brief bout of the flu halfway through the program slowed down his gains for a short time. By the end of the program, he found that when he felt unusual or unexpected bodily sensations, he was able to quickly counter his thoughts that he was having a major medical emergency. Jacob has gotten back to exercising regularly, and said that having his heart beating rapidly after a good workout no longer scares him. He reported that he hadn't had any full panic attacks since working through the program, although he did admit that it was difficult not to assume the worst while he had the flu.

Bindi worked through this program with the help of a therapist. The thoughts she was having about life not being worth it anymore scared her, so she made an appointment at the counseling center at her university. At first, even talking to the therapist was terrifying, but it got easier each time. Using the skills in this book, her therapist gradually encouraged Bindi to start interacting with her classmates. Just like speaking with her therapist, talking with classmates got easier and easier the more she did it. She developed a small but very close group of friends that she spent a lot of time with, and 4 years later she graduated from college with a degree in accounting and decided to stay in the city to take a job at a local company. She hasn't had any episodes of depression since.

Like Bindi, Jacqui chose to work through the program with the help of a therapist. She was initially concerned about seeking professional help because she worried that child protective services might be called and take her daughter away from her. This didn't happen, of course, and Jacqui was able to make great strides in reducing her fears of harming her child. She mentioned that she was able to start to understand that the horrible images that popped into her mind were just thoughts. They didn't mean that she would, or even might, harm her child. They were just thoughts. And when she stopped fighting these thoughts and fears, they mostly stopped popping into her mind. Jacqui and her partner have since had another child, a healthy baby boy, and are thinking about a third.

Through no fault of your own, anxiety has been telling you what you can and can't do. It has closed doors and restricted the pleasure you experience every day. It has taken away important parts of your life. *Turn the page and begin to take back your life.*

THE PREP

In Part I of the book, you will learn about what anxiety is and how it can become a problem for so many people (Chapter 1). You'll also take stock of how your own anxiety manifests itself (Chapter 2) and then get yourself ready to begin the program (Chapter 3). Finally, you will take the information that you identified in Chapter 2 and use it in Chapter 4 to map out the best strategies to use throughout the program, to maximize the changes that you hope to see.

As this is a workbook, we hope you will fill out all the forms as you work through "The Prep" because you will come back to them throughout the program. Take your time to make sure you understand your anxiety and how best to use the program, and then when you are ready, you can move on to Part II and begin making changes.

1

anxiety
the big picture

You're one of the millions of people who have an anxiety-related problem, but with the right help you can overcome it. You've taken an important step by beginning this book. Maybe you already know a lot about the different kinds of anxiety and have already been diagnosed with a specific anxiety disorder. Or maybe all these terms will be new to you. Either way, before you start *The Anti-Anxiety Program,* it's a good idea to build a general understanding of just what anxiety is and how it can be tamed.

Just as someone with heart disease or high blood pressure needs to comprehend the nature of the illness and get the right medical help, you need to get on the right track to rid yourself of the burden you've been carrying that has kept you from being the person you want to be—at home, at work, and in social situations. This chapter gives you a good grasp of the fundamentals: the nature of anxiety, the main types of anxiety disorders, the triggers for anxiety, its causes, and its effective treatments. We offer a few prompts to start thinking about how your own experience with anxiety fits in with this information. In the next chapter, we'll help you apply your new understanding to get a more complete picture of your particular anxiety.

Let's start with the concept that anxiety is a universal emotion experienced by everyone everywhere—probably even by most animals. We need our anxiety. It does us a lot of good in many situations. But when it's out of our control—as you know all too well—it does us harm. In fact, as hard as it may be to believe, the anxiety and fear systems in your body are probably working in exactly the way they were designed to work. They are just going off at the wrong times, just like when the smoke detector in your home sometimes goes off when you are cooking. So what *is* the function of anxiety in our lives?

What Is Anxiety?

Anxiety occurs when you're confronted with a possible threat, danger, or negative event, particularly something over which you have little control. When you feel anxious, your body becomes aroused. You may experience muscle tension, increased heart rate, and other physical changes. Your attention also becomes more focused—on the possible source of the threat as well as on your own functioning (for example, on your feelings of arousal). This process is designed to help you prevent or avoid possible danger in the future.

This focus of attention on the potential source of danger is called *hypervigilance*. Hypervigilance makes it hard for you to concentrate on your work or on other normal activities such as reading or having a conversation. You may also start to *worry*, which involves trying to think about possible plans or solutions to disarm the perceived threat. Finally, anxiety is often associated with *avoidance*. When you're anxious, you may try to avoid situations that you perceive as threatening. You may also try to avoid your own experiences—in particular, the physical sensations and anxiety-provoking thoughts that accompany your negative emotions.

Valerie, who you met in the Introduction, illustrates what happens to us when we feel anxious. She is preparing for a meeting the next day at work while her husband, Carl, is out of town on a short business trip. She begins to worry about terrible things that might happen to Carl, and her anxiety level gets very high—so high, in fact, that she can't concentrate on preparations for tomorrow's meeting. She can't help focusing on how uncomfortable she feels and whether Carl is safe.

She tries to think of ways to concentrate better, but she simply can't. Finally, she gives up, pours herself a drink, and decides to go to bed. She figures that at least she'll be well rested if not well prepared for the meeting. Unfortunately, the more she tries to fall asleep, the more aroused and awake she feels. No attempt to distract herself from her anxiety works. So she pours herself another couple drinks and hopes that she isn't hung over tomorrow at her meeting.

Clearly, Valerie is experiencing anxiety—a negative emotion focused on the possibility of future threat (in this case, bad things happening to Carl). The good news is that the strategies described in this book have helped countless individuals just like Valerie overcome their anxiety and get on with their lives.

Anxiety versus Fear

Unlike anxiety, which is focused on some *future* threat, fear is an intense emotional reaction to some *immediate* threat or danger. Helen fears snakes, for example, and experiences anxiety about possibly encountering one whenever she goes to the pet store to pick up food for her hamster. One day she actually saw a snake at the pet store, which triggered fear—her entire behavior was focused on getting out of the store as quickly as possible. Anxiety zeroes in on possible future dangers, while fear is focused on the here and now. It deals with immediate and real dangers, as well as with perceived dangers that only seem immediate and real.

Fear is the sort of response you might experience if a growling dog were chasing you, if you were being mugged at gunpoint, or if you were traveling in a car with a reckless driver, narrowly dodging one serious accident after another. When you're afraid, your body becomes mobilized for action. Your heart may start to race or pound. Your breathing rate increases. You may also experience sweating, dizziness, and many other symptoms of arousal.

Fear is also associated with a strong urge to perform some action to reduce the potential threat. That urge arises because fear activates your somatic nervous system to prepare you to face danger. Your body's response to immediate danger is often referred to as the "fight-or-flight response" because all the changes in your body are designed to help you respond to the threat with either aggression (fight) or escape (flight). In some cases, particularly in response to traumatic events, people may experience more of a "freezing" response—like a deer in the headlights. For this reason, the term "fight, flight, or freeze response" is sometimes used to describe the response to perceived threat. Most often, the action that people with anxiety problems take in response to a perceived threat involves escape, avoidance, or engaging in some sort of safety behavior to ward it off—"flight." That's why this book focuses mostly on the "flight" side of the fight-or-flight response.

> **Anxiety is a response to perceived future threats.**
>
> *Fear* **is a response to perceived immediate threat.**

The Relationship between Fear and Anxiety

We all feel fear and anxiety from time to time. But if you have an anxiety disorder, you feel these emotions frequently. You may find that you have difficulty labeling your own emotions or that terms such as *anxiety* and *fear* don't seem to capture what you feel. What terms do you use to describe the feelings that led you to start reading this book? Perhaps more general terms such as *discomfort* or *uneasiness* seem closer to what you experience. States such as terror or panic are probably more closely related to fear. Apprehension, nervousness, and worry are probably more closely related to anxiety. Pick the descriptions that seem right to you. Regardless of what words you use to describe these states, the strategies in this book can help you overcome them.

The Benefits of Anxiety and Fear

You may be surprised to learn that anxiety and fear serve a useful function. Surely you find anxiety and fear unpleasant, but you wouldn't want to be entirely rid of them. You *need* them to survive. As you just learned, anxiety is designed to help you prepare for a *possible* future threat; fear is designed to help you protect yourself in the face of some *immediate* threat. Just as you might adjust the sensitivity of the smoke detector so that it stops blaring when you are cooking, your goal here is to adjust your anxiety and fear so that they turn on only when they're appropriate to the situation.

The relationship between anxiety and performance is complex. People often assume that anxiety leads to impaired performance at work, at school, and in other activities, but it's not that simple. In fact, at low levels, anxiety has exactly the opposite effect, actually seeming to improve functioning and performance. Think about it. Many of the things you do on a day-to-day basis are inspired by your concern about the possible consequences of *not* doing these things; in other words, they're motivated by anxiety. You drive within the speed limit to avoid getting a ticket or being in an accident; you arrive at work on time each day to avoid being fired; you pay your bills to avoid the potential legal and financial consequences of not paying them.

Low to moderate levels of anxiety actually provide you with the motivation to get things done. If you had no anxiety, chances are that many necessary tasks would never be completed. You might even be inclined to do things that are impulsive and risky. For example, there is evidence that some people who engage in antisocial behavior (for example, criminal activity) may respond to particular threatening situations with less anxiety and fear than people who are not inclined toward antisocial behavior. It may be that anxiety about getting caught contributes to preventing some people from committing crimes.

Although low to moderate levels of anxiety motivate us to work hard and perform well, high levels can interfere with our ability to get things done. If you're making a big presentation at work, a moderate level of anxiety might keep you on your toes. But extreme anxiety would make it difficult for you to concentrate, thereby increasing the chances that you would lose your train of thought and botch parts of your presentation. The goal of this book, then, is not to rid you of all anxiety but to help you achieve levels of anxiety that enhance your performance, rather than get in its way.

Like anxiety, fear also has important benefits. Fear is designed to protect you from immediate danger. When you feel fear, your body goes into overdrive. Your heart rate increases to push more blood to your large muscles to facilitate escape (or fighting back); your breathing rate increases to provide the extra oxygen your body needs to flee the situation or fight off an aggressor; you sweat heavily to cool off your body so you can perform more efficiently. In fact, most of your body's responses during fear or panic make it easier for you to escape. Not only are the symptoms of fear and panic not dangerous (contrary to what many people believe when they are experiencing panic), but they are doing vital work to protect you from danger. Fear and panic are a problem only when they occur too frequently, too intensely, and in the absence of true danger, thereby preventing you from doing things that you want to do.

What Triggers Anxiety and Fear?

Anxiety and fear are reactions to perceived threat. This means essentially that we *interpret* a situation to be dangerous in some way. It doesn't mean that the situation *is* dangerous. Scary movies are a good example of this. We often feel afraid during the movie because it seems so realistic, but we aren't in any real danger of Hannibal Lecter coming out of the television and attacking us.

Anxiety and fear are almost always triggered by something. There are two main types of triggers: external and internal.

External Triggers

External triggers are objects, situations, or activities that we experience as threatening. For example, people with phobias may experience triggers in the form of heights, spiders, snakes, driving, flying, public speaking, or other things or situations. People who worry too much may become anxious when a loved one is late arriving home (like Valerie worrying about her husband). People with concerns about germs may respond to triggers such as touching elevator buttons, doorknobs, or other objects in public places. People who fear slipping on the ice may avoid going out at all on very cold days.

In all these examples, the anxiety trigger is something external to the individual. It's a place or situation (for example, a high mountain), an activity (such as sitting on a public toilet), or an object (like a dog). If you believe an external trigger poses a threat, you're likely to deal with it through *avoidance* (turning down an invitation to a party because of anxiety in social situations), *escape* (leaving a party early due to anxiety), or *safety behaviors* (wearing extra makeup and a turtleneck sweater to a party to hide blushing on your face and neck).

Internal Triggers

Internal triggers for anxiety and fear are private, internal experiences that we experience as threatening. One type of internal trigger involves physical sensations and feelings (sometimes called *interoceptive* cues or triggers). Here are some examples in which these triggers play an important role:

- A woman with panic attacks is terrified that her racing heart could cause a heart attack. She panics whenever she notices the slightest increase in her heart rate even if she knows it's caused by something else, like exercise.
- A person with claustrophobia fears suffocating in enclosed places. The sensation of breathlessness triggers a panicky feeling, particularly when she feels closed in.
- A man with a fear of heights is terrified of feeling dizzy in high places, convinced that he will lose his balance and fall.
- Someone who is nervous in social situations is particularly frightened of having shaky hands. He's convinced that other people will notice his shakiness and view him as weak or incompetent.

Another type of internal trigger involves thoughts or imagery, often referred to as *cognitive* triggers (the word *cognitive* refers to mental processes such as thinking, memory, and attention). Just as people can be afraid of their physical sensations, they can fear their own mental experiences such as thoughts, images, or urges. Consider these examples:

- A woman who was raped 5 years ago is still terrified when she thinks about that horrible event. She does everything she can to block the memories from entering her mind. She believes that if she allows herself to think about the rape, she may become so anxious that she will "go crazy" or lose control.
- A person with obsessive–compulsive disorder (OCD) is terrified of having thoughts about hurting his loved ones, especially when such thoughts pop into his head unexpectedly. He knows he won't act on these thoughts, yet he feels compelled to keep them from entering his mind.
- A man who is fearful of vomiting does everything he can to avoid thinking of vomiting. Even the thought of vomiting arouses some nausea, and he fears that thinking about vomiting could cause it to happen.

People who react to internal triggers with fear and anxiety are often afraid of their emotions, particularly of feeling anxious or frightened, which is associated with the very sensations, thoughts, and images that they view as threatening or dangerous. Note that the distinction between external and internal triggers is not always clear-cut. As you may have noticed, many of the examples of internal triggers you just read are anxiety provoking only in the context of an external situation. For example, someone with social anxiety may be frightened by feeling shaky or sweaty, but only if there are other people around to notice.

Similarly, someone with a fear of driving may fear being dizzy, but only when behind the wheel of a car. For some people, internal triggers may be anxiety provoking only in the context of particular external triggers. For others, experiencing particular sensations or thoughts may be scary no matter where or when they occur.

> *Do I have internal triggers, external triggers, or both?*

The Anxiety Disorders

As we've said, anxiety and fear are normal emotions that we all experience from time to time. Sometimes our anxiety and fear are realistic in the context, but often our reactions reflect unrealistic or exaggerated concerns. Almost everyone misinterprets events at times, so it's perfectly normal to experience unrealistic fear and anxiety on occasion. But if you experience exaggerated levels of anxiety and fear frequently, and the anxiety is causing problems in your day-to-day life, you may be experiencing an anxiety disorder. The American Psychiatric Association publishes a guide, the *Diagnostic and Statistical Manual of Mental Disorders*—currently in its fifth edition (DSM-5)—for diagnosing psychological problems, including anxiety disorders and other disorders that involve anxiety.

> *Has a mental health professional ever given me a diagnosis?*

DSM-5 lists 10 different anxiety disorders and provides specific criteria that health care professionals can use to decide whether an individual is suffering from one. In addition, in developing DSM-5, the American Psychiatric Association made a controversial decision to move trauma-related disorders (such as posttraumatic stress disorder, or PTSD), as well as obsessive–compulsive and related disorders (like OCD), out of the category of anxiety disorders, even though anxiety and fear are cardinal features of both PTSD and OCD and both of these problems respond to treatments similar to those effective for other anxiety-related problems. In this book, we continue to consider PTSD and OCD alongside the anxiety disorders.

On the following pages are descriptions of the most common ways in which people experience anxiety problems. In addition to these key features, an individual must experience significant distress about having the problem, or the problem must interfere with the individual's day-to-day life, to be diagnosed with an anxiety-related disorder. The process of diagnosing anxiety disorders or other problems is complex and requires extensive training. Sometimes even trained professionals can't agree on the best diagnosis to describe a particular person's problems. Although the information in this section will provide you with some clues regarding the types of problems you may be experiencing, it's best to be diagnosed by a professional who is experienced in assessing and diagnosing anxiety disorders. We recommend that you read through the following descriptions just to get a sense of whether you identify with any of the disorders, not to try to pigeonhole your experience of anxiety—for reasons we'll explain following the descriptions.

Panic Attack

A panic attack in itself is not actually an anxiety disorder, but it can be a feature of any of the anxiety disorders. Panic attacks also can occur in the context of other psychological problems. Moreover, many people without any particular psychological disorder experience panic attacks from time to time. A panic attack is an episode of intense fear or discomfort that comes on quickly and includes a number of physical sensations or other symptoms such as racing or pounding heart, sweating, trembling or shaking, shortness of breath or smothering sensations, choking feelings, chest pain or discomfort, nausea or abdominal discomfort, feelings of dizziness, lightheadedness, unsteadiness, or faintness, feelings of unreality or detachment, numbness or tingling sensations, and hot flushes or chills. Panic attacks are often accompanied by fear of losing control, going crazy, or dying.

To be considered a panic attack, the episode must peak within minutes; in fact, many reach their high point within seconds. Panic attacks tend to last anywhere from a few minutes to an hour or so, though they often dissipate more quickly when a person escapes from the threat. Often, panic attacks are triggered by some external situation—snakes, heights, driving, public speaking—but they can also be cued by an internal trigger, such as a feared sensation, thought, or image. Some panic attacks appear to occur out of the blue, without any obvious trigger or cue.

Panic Disorder

People with panic disorder experience panic attacks out of the blue, without any trigger or cause (at least not that they are aware of). In addition, perhaps more than any other anxiety disorder, panic disorder is associated with an extreme fear of itself—a fear of having panic attacks and the physical sensations that occur during panic. People with panic disorder tend to worry about when their next attack will happen. They also worry about possible consequences of their attacks. For example, they may worry that they're having a heart attack or stroke or that they may die, go crazy, lose control, vomit, have diarrhea, faint, or embarrass themselves in some way.

Because of these fears, people with panic disorder often alter their behavior to protect themselves from panicking or from suffering any dire consequences as a result of panic. For example, they may avoid situations in which the attacks occur or rely on "safety" behaviors such as carrying anti-anxiety medications in case a panic attack occurs, always being accompanied by someone who makes them feel safe, like a spouse or a close friend, carrying water to protect against a dry mouth, frequently checking blood pressure or heart rate, always staying near exits in public places, or driving with the window open for fear of not having enough fresh air.

Agoraphobia

Agoraphobia is a fear of being in places where escape might be difficult or where help might not be available in the event of a panic attack or panic-like symptoms. People with agoraphobia are often afraid of crowded and public places, as well as of many other situations that may arouse fear, such as driving (particularly in busy traffic, on highways, and on the inside lane), public transportation (including airplanes, buses, subways, boats, and trains), crowded places (including sports venues, malls, supermarkets, museums, busy streets, theaters, classrooms, and the like), situations from which escape is difficult (such as long lines, hair salons, dentists' offices, business meetings, parties, and bridges), enclosed places (such as small rooms, doctors' offices, tunnels, elevators, and parking garages), being alone, being far from home, or situations that trigger physical arousal symptoms (such as sex, exercise, and scary movies).

Social Anxiety Disorder

Social anxiety disorder (SAD), also known as social phobia, is an extreme fear of situations in which a person might be observed, judged, or scrutinized. People with SAD are overly concerned about being embarrassed or humiliated or making a bad impression on others. They tend to avoid situations involving direct interactions with others (interpersonal situations) and situations where they might be the center of attention (performance situations). Examples of *interpersonal situations* that are often feared by people with SAD include initiating or maintaining conversations, dating, being assertive, talking to people in authority, or attending parties, meetings, or other social gatherings. Examples of *performance situations* that are often feared by people with SAD include speaking in front of groups, eating or drinking in front of others, writing in front of others, being seen in public, making mistakes in public, working out in a gym with others around, performing in public (for example, playing music, singing, acting), or having their picture taken. The problem must be present for at least 6 months to be diagnosed as SAD.

Specific Phobia

Specific phobia refers to an excessive or unrealistic fear of a specific object or situation. Like other anxiety-related disorders, specific phobias are not diagnosed unless the fear interferes with the individual's life or is experienced as a problem, and it must also last for half a year or longer. For example, if you're terrified of snakes but you live in an area where there aren't any snakes, you would not be considered to have a phobia. There are four main types of specific phobias: (1) fear of dogs, cats, mice, spiders, snakes, bugs, moths, cockroaches, birds, lizards, or other animals, (2) fear of heights, drowning, the dark, or other aspects of nature, (3) fear of the sight of blood, watching surgery, receiving a shot, having blood tests, or having dental procedures, and (4) fear of flying, driving, being in enclosed spaces, or other particular situations. Other phobias that don't fit neatly into these types include, for example, fear of clowns.

Generalized Anxiety Disorder

People with generalized anxiety disorder (GAD) are worriers. They worry about a wide range of topics: work, school, their family, their health, money, the world, and minor matters that arise from day to day. What distinguishes the kind of worrying that would lead a person to be diagnosed with GAD? First, it needs to have been a long-standing problem—for at least half a year. Many people with GAD describe themselves as having been worriers for as long as they can remember. Second, the worry must be about many different things, not just about, say, work. Third, the worry must be excessive, out of proportion to the actual situation. Worrying about your elderly father who is being treated for a serious illness would not be excessive. Fourth, the excessive worry must be frequent—occurring on most days. People with GAD also experience other feelings, like being restless or "wired," having difficulty concentrating, carrying tension in their muscles, sleep problems, irritability, and feeling tired.

Separation Anxiety Disorder

The core feature of separation anxiety disorder is a fear of separation from home or from key figures in a person's life. This disorder is usually diagnosed in children, though it can persist into adulthood. Examples of features often associated with this problem include excessive anxiety when away from home or from parents or other caregivers; worry about losing, or harm coming to, parents or caregivers; worry that some negative event (for example, being abducted) will lead to separation; not wanting to go places like school because of separation; excessive fear of being alone, even at home; a fear of going to sleep without parents or caregivers close by (for example, a fear of sleepovers); nightmares about being separated from loved ones; or uncomfortable physical symptoms whenever separation occurs or is expected. Separation anxiety disorder always begins in childhood.

Selective Mutism

Selective mutism is almost always seen in children. It involves the inability or unwillingness to speak in situations where speaking would be expected (such as in school) despite the child's being able to speak in other situations. Little is known about selective mutism, but it appears to be related to extreme shyness or fears of embarrassment. Children with selective mutism are commonly also diagnosed with social anxiety disorder.

Substance- or Medication-Induced Anxiety Disorder

Substance- or medication-induced anxiety disorder is diagnosed when a person experiences anxiety or panic attacks immediately or soon after exposure to a substance that is capable of causing these symptoms. For example, certain stimulant medications could cause experiences of anxiety or panic. Alternatively, the anxiety or panic could come after withdrawal from the medication or substance. There needs to be no history of these symptoms before the substance or medication use.

Anxiety Disorder Due to Another Medical Condition

Other anxiety disorders are diagnosed only after the direct effects of a medical illness are ruled out. The exception is anxiety disorder due to a general medical condition, where the anxiety symptoms are due entirely to a medical illness. OCD symptoms might be triggered by a brain tumor, for instance, or panic attacks might be triggered by an overactive thyroid. If the anxiety continues after the medical illness has been treated successfully, then diagnosis of another anxiety disorder may be appropriate.

Note that medical problems can sometimes make an underlying anxiety disorder worse, though not be completely responsible for it. For example, someone with panic disorder who also has asthma may experience more severe panic attacks. Such cases would not be diagnosed in this category.

Posttraumatic Stress Disorder and Acute Stress Disorder

PTSD is an anxiety-related disorder that begins following a serious trauma in which a person's life or physical well-being is threatened, including sexual abuse, assault, or rape; physical abuse or assault; being a victim of armed robbery; serious accidents at work, at home, while driving, or elsewhere; combat; seeing someone get killed or badly hurt; or surviving a fire, earthquake, serious storm, or other disaster. During the trauma, the individual's response is one of fear, helplessness, or horror.

People with PTSD develop symptoms including (1) mentally reexperiencing the trauma, such as through repeated disturbing memories of the trauma, nightmares about it, flashbacks in which it feels as though the trauma is happening again, or becoming very upset and anxious upon being reminded of the trauma; (2) avoidance of reminders of the trauma, such as a tendency to avoid thoughts, feelings, conversations, activities, people, and places that remind the individual of the trauma; (3) changes in thinking or mood related to the trauma, such as negative beliefs about oneself, others, or the world, unrealistic beliefs about the causes or consequences of the trauma, or persistent negative emotions (for example, fear, anger, guilt, or shame); and (4) changes in arousal and reactivity related to the trauma. These include such things as difficulty sleeping, irritability, trouble concentrating, always having to be on guard for possible danger, and being startled easily.

A diagnosis of PTSD requires that the symptoms be present for at least 1 month. In contrast, a diagnosis of acute stress disorder requires many of the same symptoms but for a shorter period (lasting anywhere from 3 days to 4 weeks). In many cases, people may receive a diagnosis of acute stress disorder after a trauma and then see it changed to PTSD if the problems continue after a month.

Obsessive–Compulsive Disorder

Obsessions are irrational thoughts, images, or urges that a person has frequently and that are experienced as intrusive, inappropriate, upsetting, distressing, or frightening. Common obsessions include aggressive obsessions, obsessions about contamination, symmetry and exactness obsessions, somatic obsessions (obsessions related to the body), religious obsessions, or sexual obsessions. *Compulsions* are behaviors that people use to reduce the anxiety caused by their obsessions. These activities may follow a rigid, self-imposed set of rules that the person believes will prevent bad things from happening. Whereas obsessions tend to make people more uncomfortable and anxious, compulsions reduce their anxiety and discomfort. Examples of common compulsions include frequent checking, washing and cleaning, repeating a behavior or thought, ordering or arranging, or counting things over and over again.

Many people have doubts about whether they locked the door, concerns about contamination, even occasional thoughts about hurting a loved one. In fact, one study found that consumers were less likely to purchase a product in a store if they believed it had been touched by someone else, even if they didn't actually see another person touch the product. Does this mean that everyone has OCD? Not at all. A diagnosis of OCD requires that the obsessions and compulsions lead to significant interference, that they bother the person, or that they take up at least an hour every day.

Illness Anxiety Disorder

Illness anxiety disorder is a problem in which people have high levels of anxiety about their health, despite having no symptoms or only mild symptoms. People with illness anxiety disorder tend to engage in excessive health-related behaviors (for example, checking their body for signs of illness, seeking frequent reassurance about their health), or they may avoid health-related situations (for example, never visiting the doctor or a hospital). The problem must be present for at least 6 months to be assigned this diagnosis. Illness anxiety disorder shares features with panic disorder (for example, a fear of bodily sensations), as well as with GAD (a tendency to worry about health) and OCD (a tendency to check excessively and ask for reassurance).

Other Anxiety-Related Problems

A number of other problems often have anxiety as a core feature. The strategies in this book are often helpful for these other anxiety-related problems too.

Obsessive–Compulsive Personality Disorder

Obsessive–compulsive personality disorder (OCPD) is a problem in which people are preoccupied with orderliness, perfectionism, and a need to be in control. People with OCPD tend to be overly concerned with details, rules, schedules, lists, and organization to the point that it is difficult for them to complete tasks; the original purpose of the activity often gets buried in a mountain of detail. People with OCPD often have difficulty delegating tasks to other people and are frequently described as overconscientious and rigid. OCPD is often driven by anxiety-related beliefs that giving up control will lead to chaos in one's life. It can be difficult to distinguish it from some types of OCD; indeed, the two problems often co-occur.

Body Dysmorphic Disorder (Imagined Ugliness)

In body dysmorphic disorder (BDD), the core feature is an imagined defect in appearance. A person with a BDD may be preoccupied with thoughts of having a big nose, an asymmetrical face, or funny-shaped legs, which others don't see. People with BDD often think constantly about their "defect," taking great pains to hide it from others and checking frequently to make sure it stays hidden. BDD shares features with other anxiety-related disorders such as social anxiety disorder (for example, a fear of being observed by others) and OCD (for example, excessive checking).

Fear of Death

It's normal to fear death, and most of us do. As with any anxiety problem, it's a concern only if the fear causes you significant distress or interferes with your life. Fear of death is often a feature of another anxiety disorder. For example, people with panic disorder may worry about dying during a panic attack, people with GAD may worry about dying in general, and some people with OCD may ruminate about dying after coming into contact with some sort of contaminant that they view as dangerous. But excessive fear of death can also occur in the absence of another anxiety disorder.

Test Anxiety

Anxiety about exams or tests is another problem for which the strategies in this book may be useful. As with death anxiety, it may be a feature of another anxiety disorder. People with panic disorder may be nervous about exams, fearing they may panic and be unable to leave the exam room. People with social anxiety may worry about being judged or evaluated if they do poorly on an exam and will be particularly anxious about oral exams and presentations. People with OCD may fear tests because of a concern about making mistakes and the need to check their work over and over. People with GAD may worry about tests and exams because they worry about almost everything. Test anxiety can also exist in the absence of any other specific anxiety-based problem. For example, people with poor study skills who tend to get low grades may have realistic anxiety about tests.

Distinguishing among Anxiety-Based Problems

Did you identify with any of the disorders described on the previous page? Or did some of the features of several disorders feel familiar? If you ended up feeling somewhat confused about which description fits you, you're not alone. An anxiety problem may share features of several disorders while not meeting all the criteria of any specific one. And the features of the various anxiety problems overlap. For example, anxiety in social situations can occur across most of the anxiety disorders. People with social anxiety may be fearful of looking foolish in front of other people; people with OCD may be anxious that others will notice them repeatedly counting things or washing their hands. Similarly, a fear of flying can occur for many reasons: in panic disorder and agoraphobia, a person may fear panicking and not being able to escape from the plane; in a specific phobia, a person may fear a plane crash; in social anxiety disorder, a person may fear having to talk to the person in the next seat.

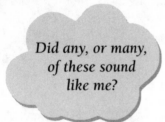

Did any, or many, of these sound like me?

A psychologist or psychiatrist could have just as much trouble as you are trying to assign a specific disorder label to your experience with anxiety. So, while it's useful to know the diagnostic terms that a professional may use if you're being evaluated for anxiety, we, like many other practitioners and scientists, now question how useful each of the specific diagnoses is.

Just because one person has anxiety around germs (possibly OCD), another has anxiety about public speaking (social anxiety disorder), and a third has anxiety about snakes (specific phobia) doesn't mean that they all have different problems. Nor does it mean that one person with all of these fears has three different things wrong. In fact, most people with one anxiety disorder also experience features of other anxiety disorders, as well as different problems, like depression. Therefore, we generally take what is often called a *transdiagnostic* view of anxiety and emotional disorders.

Transdiagnostic simply means "cutting across diagnoses." Researchers and scientists have been finding more and more evidence that the different anxiety-related disorders (as well as depressive disorders) have far more commonalities than differences. They share many of the same symptoms, are influenced by the same genetic factors, involve some of the same brain regions and neurochemicals, and are associated with the same general types of early life experiences. And most importantly, we typically use the same treatments, whether CBT or medications, for all of these diagnoses. The methods described in this book are designed to be used for symptoms of anxiety and fear regardless of the particular anxiety disorder or disorders. This is important because for many people anxiety disorders occur in clusters.

Causes of Anxiety and Anxiety-Related Disorders

Anxiety and anxiety-related disorders do not spring from any one cause. Rather, many different variables seem to influence who develops an anxiety problem and what sort of anxiety problem he develops: biological factors, psychological factors, lifestyle factors, and societal and cultural factors, among others. Of course, it's often impossible to know which factors are responsible for any one person's anxiety problem. Fortunately, we don't need to understand the cause of a person's anxiety to develop an effective treatment plan.

Biological Influences

Our knowledge about the effects of biology on the development and course of anxiety-based problems comes from research studies on genetics, brain chemistry, and specific areas of the brain that may be involved in anxiety.

Inheriting Anxiety

To some extent, we inherit the tendency to be anxious or tense. Anxiety and related disorders run in families. Our genetic makeup seems to influence the transmission of anxiety-based problems from one generation to the next. Unlike traits like eye color (for which the influence of genetics is straightforward and well understood), however, the influence of genetics on the development of anxiety disorders is complex and involves many different genes. Also, genetics is only one of many different factors that contribute to the development of anxiety disorders.

One of the challenges in trying to sort out the extent to which an anxiety disorder is inherited involves separating out the effects of genetics and environment. Family members share many of the same genes, but they also share experiences. For example, siblings raised together live in the same homes, often go to the same schools, grow up during the same period, and are raised by the same parents. To tease out the effects of genetics and environment, scientists often study large groups of twins. If an anxiety problem is based entirely on genetics, the identical twin of a person suffering from an anxiety disorder should have the same anxiety disorder. If the transmission of anxiety disorders across generations is based completely on a shared environment, one might expect the frequency of anxiety disorders to be about the same in identical twins and fraternal twins of individuals with anxiety disorders, assuming they grew up in similar environments.

Neither of these scenarios seems to be the case. Having an identical twin with an anxiety-based problem does not guarantee that a person will develop an anxiety disorder. However, the rate of anxiety disorders does tend to be higher between identical twins than between fraternal twins. Some studies show a stronger influence of genetics than do others, but nevertheless, taking into account the pattern of findings across twin studies as well as other types of genetic research, there is little doubt that genetics influences the development of anxiety.

Brain Chemistry

The brain is like a chemical factory. Information is transmitted from one nerve cell to the next by chemical messengers called *neurotransmitters*. Each nerve cell (or neuron) releases small amounts of neurotransmitter, some of which triggers a reaction in the next neuron and some of which is reabsorbed by the original neuron (in a process known as *reuptake*). The effects of this process on our body depend on the type of neurotransmitter released, the amount that is produced, the amount that is reabsorbed, the sensitivity of the receptors on the receiving neuron, and the location in the brain where the process is occurring. Examples of neurotransmitters that are believed to play a role in anxiety disorders include serotonin, norepinephrine, and gamma-aminobutyric acid (GABA).

It's believed, for example, that serotonin is involved across a range of anxiety-related disorders. Medications that increase levels of serotonin in the brain are often useful for treating anxiety-related disorders. These include the selective serotonin reuptake inhibitors (SSRIs), such as paroxetine (Paxil) and fluoxetine (Prozac), as well as certain other medications. Understanding the role of neurotransmitters in anxiety disorders has been helpful for developing new medications for anxiety. But the relationship between neurotransmitters and anxiety disorders is complex and still poorly understood. We can't tell from an individual's levels of any particular neurotransmitter whether an anxiety problem is likely to be present. Nor can we test for a specific chemical imbalance and use that information to predict a person's likelihood of success with a particular medication. What we do know is (1) that when we average across many different people, medications that affect certain neurotransmitters often reduce anxiety; and (2) that there are differences in how neurotransmitters function among groups of people *with* anxiety disorders and people *without* anxiety disorders.

Brain Activity

Advances in technology have provided scientists with effective tools to measure brain activity. For example, positron emission tomography (PET) and functional magnetic resonance imaging (fMRI) are imaging techniques that allow researchers to measure patterns of blood flow in the brain, just as X-rays can be used to provide images of bones. These imaging techniques can identify areas of the brain that are more or less active in particular anxiety disorders. However, several recent studies have found that the brain scans often cannot differentiate among people with different anxiety diagnoses, and findings from brain imaging studies are often not consistent. Also, it's difficult to conclude much about the cause of an anxiety disorder based on findings from brain imaging studies because an area of increased activity in the brain may indicate something about the *cause* of a person's anxiety disorder or it may simply be an *effect* of having the anxiety disorder.

Bringing It All Together

You may have noticed that the three previous sections on biological factors were fairly nonspecific—that there weren't any genes, brain chemicals, or brain regions that seem to specifically be related to one type of anxiety versus another. In fact, the same genes, chemicals, and brain areas seem to be involved in other negative emotions as well, such as depression and anger. Our best understanding is that these factors predispose some people to experience negative emotions more frequently and intensely than others do, but then psychological and social factors—which are discussed in the following sections—shape how each person experiences anxiety or depressive problems. This also explains why many people with anxiety problems also experience other difficulties like depression or anger.

Psychological Influences

Although biological research has contributed greatly to our understanding of anxiety, we also possess a wealth of knowledge about the influence of psychological factors. Some of the most important psychological factors known to underlie anxiety disorders include the role of learning and experience, the role of one's thoughts and beliefs, and the role of one's behaviors.

Learning and Experiences

Think about some of the most memorable experiences you've had, both good and bad. These may include the breakup of a relationship, meeting a new friend, having an accident, the death of a loved one, a fantastic course that you took in school, or even a movie that changed you in some way. We are all shaped by our histories. Psychologist Stanley Rachman proposed three types of experiences through which we learn to experience anxiety and fear in response to particular objects and situations.

One is *direct experience*. That's when we learn to fear an object or situation through some sort of direct negative or traumatic experience. Some examples include:

- Learning to fear dogs after being bitten by a dog
- Learning to fear flying after enduring a very turbulent flight
- Learning to fear driving after a car accident

- Developing a fear of public speaking after being teased following a presentation
- Learning to fear eating certain foods after suffering a bout of food poisoning

Considerable evidence indicates that negative experiences can influence fear and anxiety. In the case of PTSD and acute stress disorder, a negative experience is always the trigger. But even in the other anxiety disorders, people often report a history of one or more traumatic experiences that either initially caused the anxiety or led to a worsening of it.

Rachman's second pathway to developing fear is learning through *observation*. This happens when you learn to fear a situation by watching somebody else have a negative experience or behave fearfully in a situation. This may explain how an individual's environment can contribute to the transmission of anxiety from generation to generation. For example, a child who grows up with a parent who is terrified of driving may develop his own fear of getting behind the wheel. When a situation is unfamiliar, children often take their cues from their parents before deciding whether a situation is safe or dangerous. Watching a trusted parent panic whenever he encounters a particular object or situation may teach a child to fear that object or situation as well.

Rachman's third pathway to developing fear and anxiety involves learning through *information or instruction*—in other words, learning to fear situations via material you encounter through conversations, reading, surfing the web, watching television, and other sources of information. For example, a small boy may learn to fear germs and disease if his parents frequently warn him about the dangers of coming into contact with germs. An important route of informational learning is the news. After the 9/11 terrorist attacks, many people were reluctant to fly. Several airlines around the world even ended up declaring bankruptcy; in the United States alone more than 100,000 people lost their jobs in various airline-related businesses. People's fear of flying was probably triggered by vivid images in the media. Of course, statistically speaking, flying continues to be a very safe way of traveling.

Although these three pathways explain the occurrence of fear in some cases, they don't fully explain the relationship between learning and fear. For example, many people develop problems with fear and anxiety without ever having a negative experience, watching somebody else be afraid, or hearing about the dangers associated with a situation they fear. For some people, fears seem to begin out of the blue. And many people who have these negative experiences do not develop fears. So although these pathways may contribute to the development of fears, they don't really explain why some people develop significant fears following these experiences and others don't. It's likely that other factors (such as genetic vulnerabilities, personality styles, beliefs about the experience, behavior following the experience, and the like) also play a role.

Thinking and Anxiety

Anxiety disorders are associated with negative patterns of thinking, and having negative thoughts can contribute to anxiety and fear. One of the main differences between someone who fears driving and someone who doesn't is that the former believes that the situation is threatening or dangerous. In fact, many experts hold that to experience fear in a situation the situation must be interpreted as dangerous in some way. The box on the facing page includes examples

---

Common Beliefs Associated with Anxiety Disorders

"A racing heart is a sign that I may be having a heart attack."

"It would be terrible to panic in a movie theater."

"The dog will attack me."

"The plane will crash."

"I will run out of air on the elevator."

"If I get dizzy, I will fall from a high place."

"I will make a fool of myself during the presentation."

"People find me boring."

"My boss will think I'm incompetent."

"Nobody would ever want to date me."

"If I think about hurting a loved one, it means that I'm more likely to do it."

"I need to check my work over and over because it would be a disaster to make a mistake."

"My husband is probably late because he's been in a car accident."

"It would be terrible to be late for an appointment."

"Worrying helps to prepare me for bad things that may happen."

"I need to be the perfect parent."

"If I go out alone, I will be attacked."

"People will think worse of me if they know that I was raped."

---

of thoughts, beliefs, predictions, and assumptions that may contribute to fear and anxiety in anxiety disorders.

Behavior and Anxiety

How people behave in response to their anxiety has a big effect on whether they manage to overcome it. Two types of behavior seem to be the most problematic. The first is *avoidance*. It's natural to want to avoid a situation that triggers anxiety or fear, but avoidance helps keep the anxiety alive over time. Avoiding the feared situation means you'll probably never learn that it is indeed safe, and your anxiety may never have a chance to decrease. Although avoidance helps keep your anxiety under control in the short term, it has the exact opposite effect over the long term.

Safety behaviors are a second strategy that people often use to reduce their anxiety in the short term, but, as with avoidance, they actually help the anxiety along. In fact, safety behaviors can be thought of as a more subtle form of avoidance. The compulsions that are often part of OCD can also be viewed as extreme safety behaviors. Some examples of safety behaviors include:

- Repetitive hand washing to avoid getting sick
- Using distraction to prevent panic attacks
- Wearing a turtleneck sweater or extra makeup to hide blushing
- Wearing gloves to avoid coming into contact with germs
- Carrying a gun or knife to protect against possible attackers
- Always being accompanied by someone else in public places to feel more comfortable
- Carrying anti-anxiety medication just in case the anxiety gets out of control

Societal and Cultural Influences

Anxiety disorders occur throughout the world and across cultures, but culture can influence the *content* of a person's anxiety. Many of the anxiety syndromes described in this chapter may not occur as commonly in non-Western cultures, at least not in the same form. And people in non-Western cultures often experience anxiety problems that are uncommon in the West. For example, *koro,* an anxiety disorder that occurs in some East Asian cultures, is associated with sudden and intense anxiety that the penis (or in females, the vulva and nipples) will recede into the body, possibly causing death. *Taijin kyofusho,* an anxiety-related disorder that occurs in Japan, is an intense fear that an aspect of one's body may be unpleasant, embarrassing, or offensive to others.

Even within Western cultures, the content of a person's fear may be influenced by the individual's job, religion, or other aspects of the surrounding culture or environment. For example, people with OCD who are very religious are more likely to have obsessions with religious themes than individuals with OCD who are not particularly religious.

Cultural factors may also help explain why some fears are more common in women than in men. In Western cultures, it is much more acceptable for women to express fear and anxiety than it is for men. Men may choose to hide their feelings of anxiety, or to mask them by drinking or by responding to perceived threats with an aggressive or angry response.

As discussed earlier, the news media may also have an impact on what situations we fear. People often fear the sorts of threats that the media tell us to fear: terrorism, shark attacks, tainted food, plane crashes, murder, and anthrax poisoning. Although these threats typically harm a very small minority of the population, they tend to arouse greater fear than more dangerous (and less dramatic) threats such as smoking, alcohol abuse, and obesity.

Overview of Effective Treatments

Despite all of the possible causes, the good news is that anxiety and anxiety-related disorders are among the most treatable of psychological problems. This section provides a brief overview of the treatments that will be discussed in detail throughout this book. You will notice that certain treatments are not discussed in this section—for example, hypnosis and traditional psychotherapies. That's because they haven't been studied extensively for the treatment of anxiety disorders, so their effects remain unproven.

Cognitive Therapies

As discussed earlier, anxiety is often influenced by the thoughts, predictions, and assumptions we hold about the situation we fear. Cognitive approaches to treating anxiety involve learning to identify the sorts of thoughts that contribute to your anxiety and finding ways to replace them with more realistic and balanced predictions and assumptions. The first step in this process is acknowledging that your anxious predictions are merely guesses about what might happen. Once you recognize that your anxiety-related beliefs may not be true, the next step is to consider other ways of viewing the situation, followed by a thorough examination of the evidence. Often this process leads to a shift in thinking and ultimately to a shift in anxious feelings. Cognitive strategies for changing your anxiety are discussed in Chapters 5–7.

Behavioral Therapies

Behavioral strategies focus on changing behaviors that contribute to your problems with anxiety. Primarily, these involve breaking the habits of avoidance, employing safety behaviors, and following compulsive rituals. By learning to confront the situations you fear instead of avoiding and protecting yourself from "dangers" that in reality are minimal or nonexistent, you will learn that your anxious predictions don't come true. Don't be overwhelmed by the thought of exposure to feared situations. As you will see, exposure is conducted gradually, so the fear you experience will be manageable.

And it will be well worth it. Exposure is one of the most powerful ways of overcoming fear, and the gains from exposure tend to be very long lasting. In addition to situational exposure (discussed in Chapters 8 and 9), this book includes discussions of how exposure can be used to overcome a fear of thoughts, memories, and images (Chapter 10) and how exposure to physical symptoms can be used to overcome a fear of physical sensations, like a racing heart or dizziness (Chapter 11).

Relaxation-Based Treatments

Relaxation-based strategies have been used for decades to treat anxiety-related concerns. These include exercises involving tensing and relaxing the muscles of the body, slowing down one's breathing, and imagining relaxing scenes, as described in Chapter 12. Although relaxation training is somewhat useful for a range of anxiety problems, for most anxiety disorders this approach has not been found to be as effective as treatments involving exposure or cognitive strategies. One exception is GAD, for which relaxation is among the most effective methods. People with other types of anxiety, especially anxiety focused on specific situations (for example, social anxiety) would be advised to focus on some of the other strategies.

Mindfulness- and Acceptance-Based Treatments

Since anxiety is an unpleasant emotion, it's natural to want to do whatever we can to reduce it. But efforts to fight anxiety, to distract ourselves from it, or to "make" it go away often have the opposite effect. Mindfulness involves doing the exact opposite—being aware of one's internal experiences (such as feelings and thoughts), without evaluating them or trying to control them. Mindfulness is not new—it has been used for thousands of years to deal with feelings of anxiety and stress. Only recently, though, have scientists begun to study its effectiveness in treating anxiety disorders. So far, the news is promising. Increasingly, evidence supports the use of mindfulness-based strategies for a range of anxiety-related problems. However, there is also much debate among experts about how different the new mindfulness- and acceptance-based treatments are from more established psychological treatments like CBT. As you will see throughout this book, cognitive- and exposure-based strategies also encourage people to accept their anxiety-related feelings rather than fight them. Mindfulness- and acceptance-based strategies are discussed in Chapter 13.

Medication and Biological Treatments

Two major classes of medications have been found to be effective for anxiety disorders in large numbers of studies. One is the *antidepressants* such as paroxetine (Paxil), venlafaxine (Effexor), and others. Note that these medications are called antidepressants because they were originally developed for treating depression, but they are very effective for treating most anxiety-related disorders, even for those who are not depressed. In fact, they're used for lots of other problems, including eating disorders and pain management. The *anxiolytics* or *anti-anxiety medications* are the other type of drug that proves useful for treating anxiety problems. These include benzo-diazepines, such as alprazolam (Xanax) and lorazepam (Ativan), as well as other drugs. Generally, both types of medications for anxiety are prescribed by family physicians, psychiatrists, or other physicians, though some jurisdictions also allow other professionals to prescribe them.

Certain over-the-counter herbal products may also be useful for treating anxiety-based problems, though in many cases claims regarding these products have not been backed up by adequate research. Medications and herbal products are discussed in more detail in Chapter 4.

Conclusion

Anxiety and fear are perfectly normal emotions designed to protect us from potential danger. Perceived threats that trigger anxiety can include external situations or objects, or internal experiences, such as certain physical sensations and thoughts. The sensations that occur during a panic attack can be particularly frightening. The strategies discussed in this book are likely to be useful for a wide range of problems, including panic disorder with or without agoraphobia, SAD, specific phobia, PTSD, OCD, GAD, separation anxiety, health anxiety, other anxiety-based problems, and even depression.

Anxiety-related disorders develop through a complex interaction of biological, psychological, and social factors. Genetics play a role in the development of anxiety, and specific patterns of brain chemistry are associated with anxiety-based problems. The development and maintenance of anxiety are also associated with certain types of experiences, a tendency to think in anxious ways, and a tendency to rely on avoidance and safety behaviors to cope with anxiety and fear. You can overcome anxiety by changing your patterns of thinking and behavior that have been helping it to flourish. Confronting a feared situation through exposure therapy is one of the most powerful ways of reducing its hold on you. Learning to think in a less anxious way about frightening situations is also useful for reducing anxiety, as are relaxation-, mindfulness-, and acceptance-based strategies. Finally, a variety of medications have also been found useful for treating most of the anxiety disorders. Psychological treatments and medications may be used separately or in combination, although most recommendations are to try psychological therapy (like CBT) first, before adding or switching to medications. Regardless of how you choose to work on your anxiety, however, the first step is the most important one in your journey toward ridding yourself of your excessive anxiety and fear. And starting this book is an excellent first step!

2

getting to know your anxiety

Before beginning to work on freeing yourself from your anxiety problem, you need to understand it better. In Chapter 1, you learned all about anxiety in general. In this chapter, you'll learn about *your own* anxiety. Developing your own anti-anxiety plan must take into account the specific situations and experiences that trigger your anxiety, as well as the ways in which you personally respond to these triggers. This chapter shows you how to conduct a self-assessment that is similar to the evaluation a therapist might do during your first visit. This is a critical first step because the specific treatment strategies in this workbook that you end up using will depend on what you find out here. In this chapter, you will identify:

> **Understanding your anxiety is the first step toward changing it.**

- Situations and objects that trigger your fear

- The variables that affect your fear

- Physical sensations associated with your anxiety and fear

- Anxiety-provoking thoughts and beliefs

- The ways in which you avoid external fear triggers

- Safety behaviors that you use to protect yourself from possible danger

- The extent to which you fear and avoid certain internal experiences, such as thoughts, images, or physical sensations

- Associated problems, like depression or conflict in your relationships

As a quick word of warning, in this chapter we will be asking you to fill out a fair number of forms. Some readers have reported that the lists can be a bit tedious at first, but that they really helped them understand their anxiety much better once they were finished and reviewed the lists. Often, they saw connections they hadn't recognized before. Take your time if you need to, but it is important to get a deep knowledge of your own personal brand of anxiety—your symptoms, thoughts, and ways you try to cope—before you start trying to tackle it.

What Situations and Objects Trigger Your Fear and Anxiety?

The situations and objects that trigger anxiety and fear differ from person to person. The box below through page 35 includes some examples of common situational triggers for anxiety problems. After reviewing it, generate a list of situations and objects that trigger your fear and record them in Form 2.1. You may include examples from the box, but try to come up with some others too. If you have more than one anxiety problem (for example, you might have concerns about unusual physical sensations, anxiety about talking to authority figures, and a fear

---

Common Situational Triggers for Anxiety Problems

Situations that trigger fear of having a panic attack

Being alone

Being away from home

Transportation: cars, planes, buses, trains, subways

Crowded places: restaurants, supermarkets, malls, theaters, arenas, busy streets

Enclosed places: small rooms, tunnels, elevators

Waiting: standing in line, dentists, haircuts

Arousing activities: sex, scary movies, exercise

Situations that trigger fear of humiliation or embarrassment

Interpersonal contact with others: conversations, dating, meeting new people, parties, interviews, meetings, being assertive

Being the center of attention: public speaking, performing, playing sports, writing in public, eating or drinking in front of others

Situations that trigger particular worries

Worries about money: opening bills, spending money

Worries about work: being behind on e-mails, having a meeting with the boss, a fast-approaching deadline

Worries about family: child doing poorly on a test, spouse arriving home from work, child has a cold

Worries about health: going to the doctor, reading about medical illnesses, seeing a TV show on a particular health problem, experiencing pain, eating unhealthy foods

Worries about being on time: bad traffic, leaving home without enough time to spare

Worries about not sleeping: lying in bed, drinking coffee

Situations that trigger obsessional thoughts, urges, and images

Contamination concerns: touching "contaminated" objects such as money, doorknobs, other people, elevator buttons, and other items; coming into contact with "toxins," including detergents, chemicals, gasoline, and other such products

Irrational concerns about acting aggressively: being around certain people (for example, children) if worried about acting aggressively toward them, being around objects that could be used to hurt others (for example, knives)

Fears of particular words or images: hearing feared words, seeing feared images, talking about topics that are related to feared words or images

Concerns about making mistakes: writing letters, taking tests, having conversations, or engaging in other activities in which feared mistakes may occur

Situations that trigger a fear of particular types of trauma recurring, either in reality or in memory

Sexual assault: being around men, being alone, being sexually intimate, going out at night, watching movies with violent scenes, visiting the place where the assault took place, talking about the assault

Car accident: driving, being a passenger in a car, allowing loved ones to drive or be in a car, talking about the accident, walking on the road where the accident occurred, watching movies depicting people driving fast

Combat-related trauma: being in public places, talking about the trauma, being around other war veterans, hearing loud noises such as thunder or fireworks, seeing guns

Situations where feared animals are often encountered

Dogs: seeing dogs, being close to a dog, visiting people who have dogs, touching dogs, walking in parks or around the neighborhood, visiting pet stores

Snakes: seeing snakes at the zoo, in a pet store, or in the wild; being in areas where there may be a snake; seeing snakes in photos or on television; talking about snakes

Spiders and bugs: going outside; gardening; going into basements; seeing spiders and bugs live, on film, or in photos

Situations where blood and needles may be encountered

Blood: seeing surgery, having surgery, watching childbirth, watching medical TV shows and movies, being in a hospital or doctor's office

Needles: giving blood, having a blood test, having an injection, watching a blood test or an injection, going to the dentist

Situations where other fear triggers may be encountered

Enclosed places: tunnels, small rooms, small cars, airplanes, hugging, blankets covering the head, shower stalls, basements, closets, crawl spaces, garages, windowless rooms, crowded spaces

Flying: being on airplanes

Driving: driving on highways, driving on city streets, making left-hand turns, parking, driving in high places

Heights: ladders, rooftops, tall buildings, glass elevators, looking down over a railing, balconies, stadiums, bridges, amusement park rides

Storms: thunder, lightning, rain, snow

Water: swimming in pools, lakes, or the ocean; taking baths

Vomiting: eating certain foods, not knowing where a bathroom is, being around young children, being around sick people, reading in a car, being on a boat

Choking: eating certain foods, swallowing pills

Tests and exams: taking tests, studying for tests, taking courses that include tests, enrolling in college

of dogs), list your triggers for each problem separately (Form 2.1 includes space for three different anxiety problems; use extra paper if you need more space or download and fill in the form onscreen; see the end of the Contents for information on downloading).

If you look at Sample Completed Form 2.1, you will see an example of Bindi's feared situations and objects. Bindi, the socially anxious woman who moved to the big city to go to college, noticed that the major situations she feared included talking to strangers, speaking up in classes or giving presentations, going to parties, talking to authority figures like her professors, and going out to clubs or restaurants.

What Variables Affect Your Fear?

Now that you've categorized the situations that trigger your anxiety and fear, you need to learn to recognize the specific circumstances that affect your level of fear and anxiety in these situations. If you fear driving, for example, your level of fear may depend on all sorts of factors, including the type of car you're driving, whether it's daytime or nighttime, how tired you are, and how slippery the roads are. Why is this so important to know? In Chapters 8 and 9, you'll learn about a powerful strategy to reduce fear by exposing yourself to the situations you fear; you can influence how much fear you experience during exposure therapy by changing the variables that affect your fear in the situations in which you practice your exposures.

The box on pages 37–38 includes some examples of variables that influence fear and anxiety for various types of anxiety problems. Look over the box, then generate a list of the variables that influence your fear and record them on Form 2.2. Again, you may include examples from the table, but try to come up with other examples as well. If you have more than one anxiety problem, list relevant variables for each problem (Form 2.2 includes space for three different anxiety problems, but use extra paper if that isn't enough or download and fill the form in onscreen; see the end of the Contents for information on downloading). If your anxiety problem isn't included in the box, list it on the form with its situational triggers.

When Bindi continued working through her forms, she identified several factors that made situations harder or easier. In particular, Bindi realized that it was easier if she knew the person

Situational Triggers for My Anxiety Problems

Anxiety problem	Situational triggers
1.	
2.	
3.	

SAMPLE COMPLETED FORM 2.1 *(Bindi)*

Situational Triggers for My Anxiety Problems

Anxiety problem	Situational triggers
1. Social anxiety	Talking to strangers Speaking up or presenting in class Parties Authority figures/professors Clubs/restaurants

Variables That Often Affect Fear and Anxiety Levels

Driving: right lane versus left lane, window open versus closed, alone versus accompanied, amount of traffic, distance between highway exits, type of road, whether the radio is on, night versus day, speed of traffic, whether someone is following you too closely, whether you're tired

Buses and trains: distance between your seat and the door, distance between stops

Crowded places: how crowded, how far you are from the door, alone versus accompanied

Interacting with people: age, sex, how familiar you are with them, whether they are attractive, smart, confident, successful, aggressive

Performance situations: lighting, how formal the situation is, number of people present, position (for example, standing or sitting), whether you have been drinking, how long you're stuck in the situation, the specific activity (for example, eating messy foods versus sitting quietly)

Bodily sensations: how you feel physically (for example, fatigue)

Chronic worries: whether you can get reassurance or check to make sure your worries are not true

Intrusive unwanted thoughts: whether you can get reassurance from someone else

Sexual assault: whether you're alone when leaving the house, how familiar you are with the person you're spending time with, whether it's dark or light out when going to the mall

Car accident: speed of traffic, size of your car, type of road (for example, highway versus city street), amount of traffic, weather, dark versus light

Certain animals: size of the animal, way the animal moves (fast versus slow, jerky versus smooth movements), whether the animal is restrained (for example, dog on a leash, spider in a jar), color of the animal, whether the animal looks "mean" or angry

Blood: format of the presentation of blood (for example, in a bag, in a tube, on a person, on TV)

Needles: size of the needle, location of the needle site (for example, blood test in middle of arm, injection in top of arm, finger prick blood test, dentist's needle in the mouth), environment of the exposure (for example, hospital versus home)

Enclosed places: size of space, presence of windows, temperature, stuffiness

Flying: size of plane, duration of flight, airline, weather, amount of turbulence, whether other passengers seem "dangerous"

Heights: distance from the ground, open height versus closed in (for example, balcony versus window), distance from the edge, amount of movement around you (for example, other people walking around)

Storms: severity of the storm

Water: depth of the water, natural versus man-made (for example, lake versus swimming pool)

Vomiting: type of food being eaten, amount of motion on the boat or car trip

Choking: size of the object to be swallowed (for example, large pill versus small pill), type of food being eaten (for example, steak versus pudding)

Tests and exams: familiarity of the material, amount of studying, format of the test (for example, essay versus multiple choice)

she was interacting with, but harder if she was talking to men or if she thought the person was important or "fancy" (her word for stylish and cosmopolitan-looking people), and harder if she needed to talk about something important.

What Do You Feel When Anxious or Frightened?

In all likelihood, your fear and anxiety are associated with a range of physical symptoms and sensations. When we feel anxious or frightened, we become physically aroused. The arousal may take the form of a racing or pounding heart, sweating, trembling or shaking, shortness of breath, choking feelings, tightness or discomfort in the chest, nausea or butterflies in the stomach, dizziness, unsteadiness, faintness, feelings of unreality, feeling detached as if outside your body, numbness or tingling sensations, hot flushes, chills, muscle tension or tightness, aches and pains, or visual distortions (for example, blurred vision), as well as other uncomfortable feelings.

Is it important to be aware of the sensations you experience when feeling anxious? The answer to that question depends on how concerned you are about them. If you're not concerned at all about the physical sensations of arousal, it may not be important to spend much time trying to figure out which sensations you experience. On the other hand, if you're frightened by the sensations or if you do find them very bothersome, knowing which sensations you experience will be important when you begin to use specific strategies described in later chapters to combat your reactions. If the physical symptoms of arousal frighten you, it's important to learn different ways of responding to them.

Variables That Affect My Fear and Anxiety

Anxiety problem	Variables that affect my fear and anxiety
1.	
2.	
3.	

SAMPLE COMPLETED FORM 2.2 (Bindi)

Variables That Affect My Fear and Anxiety

Anxiety problem	Variables that affect my fear and anxiety
1. Social anxiety	How well I know the person I'm talking to
	Gender (men are more difficult)
	How "fancy" I think the people are
	How "important" I think the person is
	How "important" the topic or presentation is

It will also be helpful to recognize whether you experience panic attacks in the context of the situations you fear. Panic attacks are common among most people with anxiety-based problems. Fainting is common among people who have phobias of blood or needles, for instance, but very uncommon for people with other types of anxiety problems.

Form 2.3 provides space for you to record the physical sensations you experience when feeling anxious or frightened (it provides space for physical sensations of up to three different anxiety problems; use extra paper if you need it or download and fill the form in onscreen; see the end of the Contents for information on downloading). Think about how these sensations might vary depending on the type of anxiety problem you're experiencing. You may feel your heart race when speaking in front of groups, for example, and muscle tension and headaches when worrying about your finances.

Valerie, the woman from the Introduction who worried about everything, definitely knew about physical symptoms of anxiety. She experienced them all the time. She commonly felt butterflies in her stomach and feelings of muscle tension in her neck, shoulders, and jaw. Understandably, she also felt fatigued frequently, perhaps from all of the muscle tension she was carrying.

What Are Your Anxiety-Provoking Thoughts?

Your fear and anxiety are greatly influenced by your beliefs, thoughts, assumptions, and predictions about the situations, sensations, thoughts, and images that trigger your anxiety. Chances are that when you're feeling anxious or frightened you're predicting that something negative will occur or that the situations you fear are dangerous in some way. Are you aware of your anxious thoughts? Often people have a hard time describing their thoughts and predictions because they're so quick and automatic, almost like a habit. Do your best at this early stage in your program to identify the anxious thoughts that influence your fear. In Chapter 5 you'll have an opportunity to revisit this issue in detail.

Physical Sensations Associated with My Fear and Anxiety

Anxiety problem	Physical sensations
1.	History of panic attacks? (sudden onset of fear, with four or more symptoms; see Chapter 1) Yes ❑ No ❑ History of fainting? Yes ❑ No ❑
2.	History of panic attacks? (sudden onset of fear, with four or more symptoms; see Chapter 1) Yes ❑ No ❑ History of fainting? Yes ❑ No ❑
3.	History of panic attacks? (sudden onset of fear, with four or more symptoms; see Chapter 1) Yes ❑ No ❑ History of fainting? Yes ❑ No ❑

SAMPLE COMPLETED FORM 2.3 (*Valerie*)

Physical Sensations Associated with My Fear and Anxiety

Anxiety problem	Physical sensations
1. Worrying	Muscle tension (especially in my shoulders and neck)
	Butterflies in my stomach
	Clenched jaw
	Fatigue
	History of panic attacks? (sudden onset of fear, with four or more symptoms; see Chapter 1) Yes ☐ No ☒
	History of fainting? Yes ☐ No ☒

The box below through page 44 provides examples of typical anxious thoughts that are associated with a wide range of common anxiety-based problems. Note that some of these anxious predictions have to do with an external object or situation (for example, "The dog will bite me"), whereas others reflect concern about our own beliefs (for example, "If I think about hurting my child, that means I'm likely to do it") or our own physical sensations (for example, "If my heart races too quickly, I'll drop dead of a heart attack").

Common Anxious Thoughts Associated with Anxiety Problems

"I won't be able to cope if I have a panic attack in the theater."

"I'm guaranteed to panic if I go for a drive."

"My panic attack may never end."

"I will lose control or go crazy during a panic attack."

"If my heart races too quickly, I'll drop dead of a heart attack."

"I will faint during a panic attack."

"I will vomit or lose bowel control during a panic attack."

"Panic and anxiety are signs of weakness."

"People will think I'm weak or strange if they find out about my anxiety."

"People will think there is something wrong with me if they notice my shaking, blushing, or sweating."

"It would be terrible to make a mistake in front of other people."

"It's important for everybody to like me."

"I will make a fool of myself during the presentation."

"People are very critical and judgmental."

"I am incompetent."

"I will run out of money and won't be able to care for myself."

"My children will get into trouble if I don't take steps to protect them."

"If my family members show even mild physical symptoms, it could be a sign of serious illness."

"I won't be able to cope with the stress of work or school."

"If I don't get enough sleep, I won't be able to function the next day."

"Worrying may drive me crazy."

"Worrying helps me prevent bad things from happening."

"Touching 'contaminated' objects will make me sick."

"If I think about hurting my child, that means I'm likely to do it."

"If I have a violent thought, that means I'm a bad person."

"If I have an inappropriate sexual thought, that means I'm likely to act on it."

"If I make even a small mistake, terrible things will happen."

"I can't throw anything away in case I need it later."

"If things are out of order, I will be so overwhelmed with fear and anxiety that I will not be able to function."

"If I don't take steps to protect myself, I will experience another trauma."

"I should have been able to prevent my trauma from happening in the first place."

"The world is a dangerous place."

"If I allow myself to think about my trauma, I may lose control or go completely crazy."

"The dog will bite me."

"I will drop dead from fear if I see a snake."

"The bird will sense my fear and fly toward me."

"The spider will crawl on me."

"The needle will be painful."

"I will faint if I see blood."

"I will get AIDS from a blood test."

"I won't be able to cope if I need surgery."

"I won't be able to escape from an enclosed place."

"I will run out of air and suffocate on an elevator."

"The airplane will crash or get hijacked."

"My car will crash."

"If I stand on the high balcony, it will collapse."

> "If I get dizzy in a high place, I'll fall."
>
> "In a high place, I will become overwhelmed with an urge to jump."
>
> "I will be struck by lightning during a storm."
>
> "I will drown if I go into the water."
>
> "If I vomit, the experience will be so unpleasant that I won't be able to cope."
>
> "I will choke and die if I eat meat."
>
> "I will do poorly on my exam and fail my course."

Once you have reviewed the examples in the box, complete Form 2.4 (add paper if you need space for more than three different anxiety problems or download the form and fill it in onscreen before printing; see the end of the Contents for information on downloading the form) by recording the anxiety-provoking thoughts and predictions that run through your head when you're feeling anxious or frightened. The best way to identify your anxious thoughts is to ask yourself questions like "What am I afraid will happen?" and "What would be so terrible about being in the situation I fear?"

In the Introduction you also met Jacob, the man who feared headaches because he thought they meant he might be having a stroke, just like his father did. He also started to fear having his heart start to race, as it could mean he was having a heart attack. Jacob felt that these two fears were different, so he filled out two sections of his form. For headaches, he identified the thoughts "I'm having a stroke," "I'm going to die or become disabled," and "I'm going to end up like my dad." The thoughts about his racing heart were similar. He identified "I'm having a heart attack," "I'm going to die," and "If it isn't a heart attack, I'm probably still damaging my heart."

What Situations and Objects Do You Avoid?

The urge to avoid feared situations can be very strong, maybe even overwhelming. Naturally, if you're convinced that a situation is dangerous or threatening, you'll do what you can to avoid it. What situations and objects do you avoid? The list of situations that you avoid will probably be very similar to the list of situations and objects that trigger your fear, which you recorded on Form 2.1. Having a comprehensive list of situations you avoid will be useful when you begin to plan exposure practices in Chapters 8 and 9.

Form 2.5 can be used to record the situations you tend to avoid because of your anxiety and fear, as well as how frequently you avoid each situation (add extra paper if you need to record situations for more than three different anxiety problems or download and fill in onscreen; see the end of the Contents for information on downloading). For each anxiety problem, list the situations and objects you tend to avoid in the second column (referring back to your list of anxiety triggers on Form 2.1 will be helpful). In the third column, record a number from 0 to 100 to represent how frequently you avoid each situation (0 means that you never avoid the

FORM 2.4
Thoughts Associated with My Anxiety Problems

Anxiety problem	Anxiety-provoking thoughts	How much do I believe the thought is true? (0%–100%)
1.		
2.		
3.		

SAMPLE COMPLETED FORM 2.4 *(Jacob)*
Thoughts Associated with My Anxiety Problems

Anxiety problem	Anxiety-provoking thoughts	How much do I believe the thought is true? (0%–100%)
1. Headaches	I'm having a stroke	90%
	I'm going to die or become disabled	65%
	I'm going to end up like my dad	90%
2. Heart pounding	I'm having a heart attack	80%
	I'm going to die	80%
	If it isn't a heart attack, I'm probably still damaging my heart	90%

situation; 50 means that you avoid the situation about half the time; and 100 means that you avoid the situation completely).

As Jacob continued with his forms, he initially thought that he didn't avoid many things. But as he thought more about it, he remembered that he had stopped drinking caffeinated drinks (for example, coffee or sodas) because he didn't like how they could sometimes give him a headache or speed up his heart rate. He also stopped engaging in arousing activities (for example, going to the gym or watching exciting movies or sports) because they made his heart race and stopped drinking alcohol (especially red wine) because he feared a hangover headache, and he generally tried to limit how frequently he went to places like grocery stores where they had lots of bright fluorescent lights that sometimes triggered headaches.

How Do You Protect Yourself from Danger in the Situations You Fear?

Sometimes it's impossible to avoid a situation completely, and yet the urge to self-protect is very strong. Therefore, when people are exposed to situations they fear, they often rely on safety behaviors to protect themselves. In the case of obsessive–compulsive disorder (OCD),

Situations I Avoid

Anxiety problem	Situations and objects I avoid	Frequency of avoidance (0–100)
1.		
2.		
3.		

SAMPLE COMPLETED FORM 2.5 *(Jacob)*

Situations I Avoid

Anxiety problem	Situations and objects I avoid	Frequency of avoidance (0–100)
1. Headache	Caffeine	100
	Drinking too much alcohol	80
	Drinking any red wine	100
	Places with lots of fluorescent lights, like the supermarket	50
2. Heart pounding	Vigorous exercise	70
	Caffeine	100
	Watching action movies or sports	60

compulsions such as checking, washing, cleaning, counting, and repeating are actually safety behaviors that people with OCD use to try to guard against their fears. All the anxiety disorders are associated with safety behaviors to varying degrees. The box below and on the facing page includes examples of a wide range of anxiety safety behaviors.

After looking over the examples in the box, generate a list of your own safety behaviors and record them in Form 2.6. You guessed it: you may include examples from the box, but

---

Common Safety Behaviors Used by People with Anxiety Problems

Sitting in the aisle seat in a theater to facilitate a quick escape

Always having a "safe person" around when going into feared situations

Carrying medication in case a panic attack comes on

Frequently checking your pulse to make sure your heart isn't beating too quickly

Sitting down and resting when panic feelings begin

Cleaning the house as a distraction from panic sensations

Wearing makeup to hide blushing

Wearing light clothing to hide sweating in public

Eating in dimly lit restaurants so people won't notice you blushing

Overpreparing for presentations

Avoiding certain topics of conversation

Avoiding eye contact when talking to others

Leaving home extra early for appointments so there's no chance of being late

Phoning your children frequently to make sure they're okay

Not carrying money or wearing jewelry for fear of being mugged, even in areas that most people would consider safe

Not buying things you can easily afford for fear of one day having no money

Exercising excessively to prevent possible health problems

Wearing gloves when touching things that may be "contaminated"

Excessive hand washing to clean off possible contamination

Repeated checking to make sure that work was done correctly

Engaging in superstitious behaviors to prevent bad things from happening

Making sure things are organized perfectly to avoid feeling a sense of discomfort or incompleteness

Repeating positive words or phrases to yourself to replace frightening thoughts that pop into your mind

Carrying pepper spray to protect yourself from possible assault

Driving extra slowly to avoid a possible car accident

Walking with your back to the wall in public places to prevent the possibility of being attacked from behind

Checking for dogs through the window before leaving the house to go for a walk

Carrying an umbrella or a stick to protect yourself from harmless snakes while out walking

Making sure the basement is brightly lit before going downstairs in order to see any spiders or insects that might be there

Lying down during a blood test to avoid becoming faint

Looking away during an injection

Asking the doctor to leave the examination room door open during a medical exam to avoid feeling closed in

Flying in business class to avoid feeling closed in

Driving only in the right lane to make it easy to pull over if necessary

Driving in the left lane on bridges to protect yourself from seeing over the edge

Staying in the basement with the lights on and the music turned up to avoid seeing lightning and hearing thunder during a storm

Overpreparing for tests and exams

FORM 2.6

My Safety Behaviors

Anxiety problem	Safety behaviors	Frequency of safety behavior use (0–100)
1.		
2.		
3.		

From *The Anti-Anxiety Program, Second Edition,* by Peter J. Norton and Martin M. Antony. Copyright © 2021 The Guilford Press. Purchasers of this book can photocopy and/or download additional copies of this material (see the box at the end of the Contents).

please try to come up with other examples too. If you have more than one anxiety problem, list your triggers for each problem in Form 2.6, using extra paper if needed (or downloading the form and filling it in onscreen; see the end of the Contents for information on downloading).

Jacqui, the new mom who started having anxiety-producing intrusive thoughts that she might harm her newborn daughter (see the Introduction), knew her safety behaviors very well. She generally tried to make sure her partner was with her whenever she went to check on the baby but also developed a routine of compulsively checking her daughter head to toe four times to make sure she hadn't hurt her. When she went into a new room, she would also check the room four times to make sure there weren't any dangerous objects around. If she found something, she would move it to the other side of the house and then go back and recheck the room four times.

SAMPLE COMPLETED FORM 2.6 *(Jacqui)*

My Safety Behaviors

Anxiety problem	Safety behaviors	Frequency of safety behavior use (0–100)
1. *Being alone with my baby*	*Call out for my partner to help me*	*98*
	Check four times to make sure I haven't accidentally harmed her	*100*
2. *Having dangerous objects around*	*Check room four times to make sure there is nothing dangerous*	*100*
	If I find something, I move it to the far side of the house and check four times again	*95*
3. *Driving with daughter in car*	*Usually don't*	*80*
	Drive very slowly and only on side streets	*100*
	At every stop, turn to make sure she is okay	*100*

What Internal Experiences Do You Fear and Avoid?

As described earlier, for most people anxiety problems are triggered by particular situations, such as driving, public speaking, being in high places, or confronting a feared animal. But people are also often anxious about their own private experiences, including the physical sensations they experience and the thoughts, images, urges, and memories that run through their minds.

Fear of Physical Sensations

Fear of physical sensations is very common among people with certain types of anxiety disorders. For example:

- A person with unexpected panic attacks may be fearful of sensations that may be mistaken for a heart attack (racing heart, breathlessness, sweating), being about to faint (dizziness, lightheadedness), or being about to go "crazy" or lose control (feelings of unreality, feeling detached from oneself).

- A person with social fears may be fearful of blushing, shaking, sweating, or showing other visible signs of anxiety in front of other people.

- A person with a fear of heights may be fearful of getting dizzy because it might lead to falling.

- A person who fears driving may be anxious about feeling lightheaded because it might lead to a car accident.

- A person with claustrophobia may fear that sensations of breathlessness in an enclosed place are an indication of suffocation.

In the first column of Form 2.7 is a list of physical sensations that often occur when people feel anxious or frightened, as well as for other reasons. In the second column, record how frightened you would be to experience the sensation in general (in a situation that's normally calm for you—for example, feeling dizzy while watching TV). Use any number ranging from 0 to 100, where 0 equals no fear at all and 100 equals as frightened as you can imagine being. In the third column, record a number to indicate how frightened you would be to experience the sensation in a situation that normally makes you feel anxious (for example, feeling dizzy in a high place). In later chapters, you'll learn some strategies to overcome any fear you experience in response to physical sensations. As with the preceding forms, use extra paper if needed or download the form and fill it in onscreen to fit in more (see the end of the Contents for information on downloading).

Jacob completed Form 2.7 and found several symptoms that really scared him, especially having a racing or pounding heart, chest pain, lightheadedness, tingling sensations in his finger, and blurry vision. All of these, he thought, were signs of a possible heart attack or stroke. The other feelings, like sweating, hot flushes, or being short of breath, didn't bother him much at all.

FORM 2.7

Fear of Physical Sensations

Sensation	Fear of sensation in general (0–100)	Fear of sensation when in a feared situation (0–100)
Racing or pounding heart		
Chest tightness or pain		
Dizziness, faintness, lightheadedness		
Breathlessness or smothering sensations		
Sweating		
Hot flushes or chills		
Numbness or tingling sensations		
Nausea or abdominal discomfort		
Choking feelings or a tightness in the throat		
Blurred vision		
Feeling unreal or detached		

Fear of Thoughts, Images, Urges, and Memories

Sometimes people fear their own thoughts. In other words, they respond to their own thoughts, memories, urges, and images as if they are dangerous. They may do everything they can to prevent themselves from having these thoughts, which just makes the problem worse. Examples of people who fear their thoughts include:

- A man with obsessive–compulsive concerns who worries that if he thinks about hurting a loved one, he's likely to do it
- A woman who fears that having a negative thought about God pop into her head means that she's a bad person

SAMPLE COMPLETED FORM 2.7 *(Jacob)*

Fear of Physical Sensations

Sensation	Fear of sensation in general (0–100)	Fear of sensation when in a feared situation (0–100)
Racing or pounding heart	95	100
Chest tightness or pain	90	90
Dizziness, faintness, lightheadedness	100	100
Breathlessness or smothering sensations	10	40
Sweating	10	30
Hot flushes or chills	10	25
Numbness or tingling sensations	70	70
Nausea or abdominal discomfort	0	0
Choking feelings or a tightness in the throat	0	0
Blurred vision	75	75
Feeling unreal or detached	50	75

- A person who fears that if she thinks about her worries too much, she won't be able to sleep
- A person with a driving phobia who fears that having impulses to drive off a bridge means he will act on these urges
- A person who was sexually assaulted who is afraid to allow herself to remember the rape because she might not be able to cope with the memories

On the blank lines that follow, describe any thoughts you tend to experience that you find frightening because it feels as though the thoughts themselves might be dangerous or threatening. You may also record any memories that frighten you, as well as any scary images, impulses, or urges. (If you're not afraid of these thoughts, if you make no effort to suppress them, and you don't believe that your thoughts, images, or impulses are dangerous, skip this exercise.)

_____

_____

_____

_____

_____

_____

_____

_____

Are You Experiencing Any Other Difficulties?

Now we'd like you to reflect on whether there are any other difficulties in your life that may affect your ability to work on your anxiety problem, such as other emotional problems like depression, substance use problems such as alcohol or drug abuse, medical illnesses (for example, heart disease or chronic pain), interpersonal problems like relationship difficulties, and life stresses, including a hectic work schedule or significant financial problems. Having other problems doesn't mean you shouldn't try to overcome your anxiety at this time. If the other problems are so severe or impairing that you can't imagine focusing on your anxiety right now, however, you should work on the other issues first and then come back to the anxiety.

Do I have any other difficulties right now?

In the space below, record any other difficulties that might have an effect on your ability to follow the program described in this book. Describe whether you can work around these difficulties or put them off to the side in order to work on your anxiety.

_____

_____

_____

_____

_____

_____

_____

_____

Keeping Tabs on Your Progress

The process of self-assessment is important for developing a plan up front, and it's also useful for assessing whether your plan is working down the road. You should refer back to your responses on the forms in this chapter from time to time to see how things have changed. As you work through the strategies in this book, you will find it helpful to know if your anxiety is still triggered by the same sorts of situations, feelings, and thoughts that triggered it at the start of your program. You'll also want to know whether your anxiety-related sensations, thoughts, and behaviors have changed over time and whether your anxiety interferes with your life in the same ways it did when you began to work through this book.

If you were on a plan to lose weight, chances are you might weigh yourself from time to time to keep a record of your progress. In the same way, it will be helpful to keep track of your progress in this program by completing Form 2.8. Each week (ideally on the same day), complete the two ratings across one row of this form.

Jacqui completed her weekly ratings every Sunday morning. The first week wasn't that bad, only reaching an average of about 40, but the next week was a disaster. She had to drive her daughter to the pediatrician for a checkup and had intrusive thoughts about harming her child all week. It started to get a bit better the next week, but as she progressed through her program she found that her thoughts were becoming less frequent and bothersome and she was able to take her daughter out for short drives fairly easily.

Digital Tools

As smartphones and mobile devices have become so ingrained in our lives, it's not surprising that many people using this program (and other treatments for anxiety) prefer to use apps for monitoring their anxiety week to week. In the Resources section at the end of this book we describe several apps and websites that can be helpful for monitoring your anxiety such as MoodKit, Self-Help for Anxiety Management, and Sanvello for Stress & Anxiety. Please note that we haven't evaluated the extra components in these three apps—like relaxation techniques or games that are supposed to relieve anxiety. In general, however, we believe that it's best to try one treatment program at a time, as different ones may give conflicting advice or even work against the other. In other words, feel free to use the apps for monitoring, but stick with this program to help you overcome your anxiety.

Conclusion

In this chapter, you explored all facets of your anxiety problem as a first step toward planning your anti-anxiety program. Specifically, you identified the situations, objects, sensations, and thoughts that trigger your anxiety, as well as the ways in which you respond to your anxiety-provoking triggers. You also began to monitor the severity of your anxiety problem, a process that you will continue through the program. The information you gathered in this chapter will be used as you prepare to overcome your anxiety problems in the remaining chapters in this book. Good luck!

Weekly Record of Anxiety

Date	Average overall anxiety in the past week (1–100; 0 = no anxiety, 100 = very severe anxiety)	Overall change since the beginning (–10 to +10; –10 = much worse, 0 = no change, +10 = much better)

Weekly Record of Anxiety

Date	Average overall anxiety in the past week (1–100; 0 = no anxiety, 100 = very severe anxiety)	Overall change since the beginning (–10 to +10; –10 = much worse, 0 = no change, +10 = much better)
Apr 10	40	0
Apr 17	100	–10
Apr 24	80	+5
May 1	30	+10
May 8	30	0

3

getting ready
for the program

Working through this book will give you the tools you need to confront and overcome the anxiety that has been holding you back. But it will demand something of you—it will take your full attention, your desire and willingness to change, and your time. This chapter will help you decide whether you're committed to making these changes today and get ready to take the steps to overcome your anxiety. You'll also explore the options of working through this program on your own, with the help of a close friend or family member, or with a professional therapist.

Is Now the Best Time to Start This Program?

You may feel a bit nervous about going forward with this program and worry about how you'll find the time to practice the exercises recommended in this book. That's perfectly normal. But if you feel you can't make these commitments, we advise you not to undertake the program now, as it may mean compromising the outcome or feeling disappointed or discouraged by your results. If you're ready for it, there is every reason to believe that you will experience significant improvements in your anxiety, just as most people using the strategies described in this book have.

Here are some issues to consider in deciding whether this is the best time for you to start this program: (1) the severity of your problem, (2) your level of motivation and the potential costs and benefits to you of overcoming your problem, and (3) potential obstacles and challenges to overcoming your problem.

How Much of a Problem Is Your Anxiety?

Daniel is terrified of driving, especially on highways. Because of his fear, he can't take the sorts of trips that he and his girlfriend would love to take, and he has turned down several jobs that would have required him to drive to work. He relies on public transit and on help from his friends and family to get around. Daniel is embarrassed by his fear and he wishes he could be more at ease when driving.

Nisha gets very nervous when speaking in front of groups, so she avoids public speaking at all costs. She works in customer service, so public speaking never comes up in her job. She encounters the possibility of public speaking only every few years when she is asked to make a toast or give a short speech at a party or wedding (which she always turns down). Nisha rarely thinks about her fear of public speaking, and it doesn't really bother her.

Clearly, Daniel is a better candidate for this program than Nisha. Daniel's anxiety causes a lot of problems in his personal and professional life, which means he's likely to be motivated to get help and to work hard to overcome his fear. For Nisha, however, addressing her anxiety may be a lot of work without much payoff, so it's unlikely to be a priority for her.

It's perfectly normal to feel anxious from time to time, to fear certain objects and situations, and to avoid places and situations that trigger your fear. Anxiety and fear become a problem only when they're bothersome to you or stop you from doing things that are important to you. You wouldn't be reading this book if anxiety didn't already feel like a problem to you, but knowing *how* problematic your anxiety feels can help you know whether to make the commitment to this program and motivate you to take it on. Answer the following questions:

1. How often do significant anxiety and fear come up in your day-to-day life?

    _____

    _____

2. How much does it bother you that you have difficulties with anxiety and fear?

    _____

    _____

3. In what ways do your anxiety, fear, avoidance, and safety behaviors interfere with your life, including work, school, relationships with family and friends, intimate relationships, health, hobbies and leisure activities, management of your finances, management of household responsibilities, religious expression, or other areas?

    _____

    _____

If your anxiety comes up frequently, is bothersome to you, and interferes with your life, it's time to do something about it! And you probably wouldn't have picked up this book if you didn't already know that.

What Are the Costs and Benefits of Overcoming Your Anxiety?

Over the last few decades a considerable amount of research has been looking at the effects of motivation on treatment success. Not surprisingly, people who are less motivated tend to have poorer responses to treatment and are more likely to stop before the treatment is finished. But the tricky part is that many people *think* they are fully motivated to begin treatment when they really have a fair degree of ambivalence. When we say "motivated," we mean being ready and having no ambivalence about making changes in their lives. Low motivation does not mean being lazy. It simply means that something is interfering and keeping the person from engaging in the treatment. If you're not very motivated, perhaps it's because there are other demands competing for your time and energy. Maybe we haven't explained the reasons for various parts of the program very well. Or perhaps someone else is discouraging you from moving forward.

Am I ready to fully commit to my recovery?

Fortunately, this research into motivation and treatment has led to the development of *motivational enhancement strategies* designed to help people resolve their ambivalence and boost their motivation. These strategies are often a part of a form of psychotherapy known as *motivational interviewing*. Motivational interviewing was originally designed for people who are experiencing difficulties with alcohol or drugs but now is widely used with individuals who have a range of psychological or emotional difficulties. Motivational enhancement strategies help people evaluate and weigh the pros and cons of making changes in their lives—including engaging in this treatment program—by considering them in the context of their long-term goals and desires.

It's important to understand that these strategies are not intended to coerce or trick you into working on your anxiety, or doing anything else that you're not currently motivated to do. When you go through the process of weighing the pros and cons, you might decide that you're not yet ready to start pushing yourself through this program, *and that is okay*. The book will still be here if and when things change for you. You may still be on the fence, *and that is okay too*. Or you may find that you're ready to charge into this program right now, and *that is also okay*.

Before launching into this program, you should also be aware that motivation comes and goes. You may be highly motivated now, but that can change. Maybe things in your life will get stressful and your motivation or ability to stick with the program will go down. Maybe some of the chapters will be extra difficult for you. For this reason, we have added little motivational enhancement refreshers to several of the chapters to help you weigh the pros and cons, and your long-term goals and desires, to keep your motivation as strong as it was at the start.

If overcoming your anxiety is associated with many costs and relatively few benefits, you may decide not to work on the problem right now. On the other hand, if the benefits of overcoming your anxiety outweigh the costs, then tackling the problem now may be a good idea. At the top of Form 3.1, think about and record your long-term goals and desires related to your anxiety and your life. What are some of the things you would like to be able to do in your life? How do you see your ideal life looking in 1 to 3 years?

After you've had a chance to think over some of your long-term goals, work through the four pros and cons sections on Form 3.1, listing the costs and benefits of using the program and not using the program, and rating each one you list at 0 (not important) to 100 (extremely important). This type of exercise is often called a cost–benefit analysis. Sample Completed Form 3.1 shows how Valerie, who experiences chronic worry, filled out the form.

Now that you have everything laid out in front of you, it's time to weigh the pros and cons honestly, especially in light of your long-term goals and desires. For some people it's quite easy

FORM 3.1

Costs and Benefits of Using This Program

What are your long-term goals and desires? What would you like to do with your life in the next 1 to 3 years?
_____
_____
_____
_____

Now, thinking about your own anxiety and your own life, record the costs and benefits of (1) working through this program and (2) not working through this program.

Working through the program (0–100 importance)		Not working through the program (–100–0 importance)	
Pros _____	(___)	Pros _____	(___)
_____	(___)	_____	(___)
_____	(___)	_____	(___)
_____	(___)	_____	(___)
Cons _____	(___)	Cons _____	(___)
_____	(___)	_____	(___)
_____	(___)	_____	(___)
_____	(___)	_____	(___)

to see that the pros far outweigh the cons and will help them get to their long-term goals, but for many it isn't always so clear cut. As you can see, Valerie had some concerns about trying the program (such as worrying about whether she would do it correctly) as well as some reasons in favor of not starting the program (such as believing that worrying makes her more careful). But for her, the advantages of starting (such as hopefully worrying less) and the disadvantages of not starting (especially missing a chance to be happier) were extremely important. And most of all, the potential advantages of working through the program were much more in line with her long-term goals of being calmer and more able to handle uncertainty in life.

SAMPLE COMPLETED FORM 3.1 *(Valerie)*

Costs and Benefits of Using This Program

> **What are your long-term goals and desires? What would you like to do with your life in the next 1 to 3 years?**
>
> Being a LOT calmer, feeling safe, and not worrying so damn much
>
> Able to handle uncertainty without assuming the worst
>
> Able to do things on my own without checking on Carl every 30 minutes
>
> _____
>
> **Now, thinking about your own anxiety and your own life, record the costs and benefits of (1) working through this program and (2) not working through this program.**

Working through the program (0–100 importance)		Not working through the program (–100–0 importance)	
Pros Less anxiety/worry	(95)	**Pros** Can't fail if I don't try	(50)
Less drinking to cope	(95)	Worry makes me careful	(60)
Less muscle tension	(70)	_____	( )
_____	( )	_____	( )
Cons Another thing to worry	(80)	**Cons** Miss a chance to be	(90)
about	( )	happier	( )
Take up lots of time	(80)	Carl gets tired of my	(90)
_____	( )	worries	( )

What Are the Obstacles and Challenges That May Get in the Way?

Take this opportunity to identify any obstacles that may interfere with your program and think about possible solutions. We'll discuss some common challenges, as well as ideas for overcoming them. At the end of this section you'll have an opportunity to identify obstacles that may negatively affect your own progress and to brainstorm possible solutions (see Form 3.2).

Not Enough Time to Devote to the Problem

One of the most common reasons people put off addressing their anxiety is lack of time. To get the most out of this program, you need to spend some time working on the problem almost every day—whether it's reading this book, completing various forms and worksheets, or using the strategies described in the book. The amount of time you need will depend on the types of problems you're working on, the number of different anxiety issues you have, the severity of your anxiety and related issues, and how quickly you respond to the program. Some people are able to overcome their anxiety with relatively little effort (maybe with just a few hours of a certain practice), but most people will need a few weeks or months of hard work (such as practicing for an hour or two almost every day).

Even if you feel there are too many demands on your time, you may be able to adapt the program to suit your schedule. Many of the strategies can be used at various levels of intensity, depending on the time you have available. For example, if you're using exposure-based strategies to overcome a fear of driving, you can practice driving several evenings per week for an hour or so, and chances are you will notice that you're feeling less fearful after several weeks or months. Alternatively, you can take a couple of weeks off work and make driving practice your full-time job. By practicing driving all day long for a week or two, you might notice just as much improvement as the person in the previous scenario.

You'll see that many of the strategies described in this book can be integrated into your regular routine so they don't take up extra time. Schedule your homework practices just as you would any other activities or appointments in your life. If they're written into your schedule, you'll be more likely to find the time to get them done.

Serious Stresses in Your Life

If you're currently experiencing significant ongoing stress, it may be particularly difficult to devote the energy and focus needed to overcoming your anxiety problems right now. The kind of stresses that may pose a problem include extreme work stress, such as too much work, tight deadlines, a difficult boss, the threat of losing your job, or unemployment; relationship problems like frequent arguments, a recent breakup, or an abusive relationship; family stress, such as illness, death, legal problems, or childcare issues; and other stressors such as financial hardship, upcoming exams, moving, or medical problems.

If the stress you're experiencing is short term, consider waiting to begin this program until after it has passed. But if the stress is chronic and likely to continue for a while, you may as well begin working on your anxiety now, particularly if you think you can focus on the problem despite the stress. The good news is that some of the strategies discussed in this book (particularly those in Chapters 5, 12, and 13) have the added benefit of helping you manage the stress in your life more effectively, in addition to helping with your anxiety problems.

Financial Challenges

Some of the treatment strategies discussed in this book may cost money. It may be difficult to overcome a fear of flying, for example, without practicing flying on airplanes. Similarly, overcoming a fear of eating in restaurants requires you to practice dining in public. If you decide to use this book in the context of therapy with a mental health professional, you'll also need to consider the therapist's fees (depending on your insurance coverage). If your finances are tight, you may need to limit how much you practice the exercises that aren't free or inexpensive.

FORM 3.2

Obstacles and Challenges to My Treatment

In the first column, record any obstacles or challenges that you anticipate may affect your treatment as you work through this program. In the second column, record possible ways in which you can overcome each obstacle.

Obstacle or challenge	Solution

Lack of Support or Resistance from Friends or Family

A lack of support from friends or family members can make it more difficult to overcome problems with anxiety (or any problem, for that matter). If friends and family trivialize your problems, tease you for feeling anxious, or become angry because you aren't able to do things that frighten you, these behaviors can undermine your motivation. Some of the practices described in this book work best if done with the help of a friend or family member, which will be impossible if you don't feel you can approach one for help. If this is the case, you should be reassured to know that many people are able to overcome their anxiety problems without such outside support.

If you're fortunate enough to have the help of friends or family, though, take advantage of it as you carry out the program. Have your close friends or family members who will be involved read the box on the facing page, which provides suggestions for how they can help with the treatment process. (You might want to photocopy the box to hand out, or download and print extra copies; see the end of the Contents for information.) They may also find it helpful to read other sections of this book.

Including a Helper or "Co-Therapist"

Although it's certainly not necessary to include a family member or close friend as a helper or "co-therapist," doing so may be helpful for a number of reasons. First, your helper can offer support when you feel anxious or panicky and can help to brainstorm strategies for tackling your anxiety. Also, your helper can accompany you when you start exposure practices, particularly in situations you are too frightened to enter alone. Finally, involving someone else in your therapy can provide you with an extra incentive to follow through on your homework, just as having a buddy can give you that extra bit of motivation to get yourself to exercise.

If you decide to involve someone else in your therapy, here are some qualities you should look for:

- Someone you can trust, with whom you feel comfortable discussing the details of your anxiety problem

- Someone who is empathic and understanding

- Someone who is willing to become familiar with the procedures used in this program and to read relevant parts of this book, particularly those points listed in the box on the facing page.

- Someone who will understand that *you* are in charge of your therapy and that his role is to be supportive and encouraging and not to force you to do anything that you have not agreed to do

- Someone who will not become angry or frustrated if you are unable to complete a particular practice or if you become anxious during a practice

Do I have someone who can support me through the program?

Depending on your relationship with your helper, she will be involved to a greater or a lesser extent in your program. A partner or spouse may be more inclined to read this whole book and to be highly involved in your treatment. A friend or family member, on the other hand, may be less involved and may join you only on a couple of exposure practices. You may end up deciding to involve a few different helpers so that no one person feels overly inconvenienced.

A Guide for Family and Friends

From the time we are born to the time we die, we depend on our relationships with others for just about everything: food, shelter, work, education, health care, entertainment, companionship—you name it. In our closest relationships, we have an important effect on each other's emotional lives. The positive emotions we feel sustain us and make life worth living. The negative emotions we feel, such as anxiety, depression, and anger, are often tied to what's happening in our relationships.

If you're close to someone who suffers from anxiety, you're aware that the anxiety problem affects you too. You may be less aware, though, of how your behavior can affect her anxiety and of what you can do to help this important person in your life. These tips are specifically for the family member, close friend, partner, or other significant presence in the life of someone with anxiety.

- **Learn about your loved one's anxiety and its treatment.** The single best way to help a loved one who is working on an anxiety problem is to be informed. One thing you can do is read this book to learn more about the nature and treatment of her anxiety problems. We also recommend that you invite your loved one to talk to you about her anxiety and that you participate in the discussion in a supportive, nonjudgmental way.

- **Be supportive.** Overcoming anxiety problems can be challenging. There will be ups and downs. What your loved one needs isn't a coach or a bystander but someone to help celebrate the improvements and support him when things aren't going as well.

- **Ask your loved one how you can help.** There is no single best way to help someone who is experiencing anxiety. Some people do best when their friends and family members participate in "exposure" practices. Some people find it helpful to talk through an anxiety-provoking situation to help them see their fears more realistically. Others prefer that family members and friends remind them to complete their forms or stop avoiding situations (careful, though—there's a fine line between "reminding" and "nagging"). Some may simply want someone to listen and provide support. Finally, some people may prefer that their friends and family not get involved at all. Rather than "helping" in a way that may not be helpful, ask your loved one how you can help and respect her wishes.

- **Manage your own expectations.** Seeing loved ones change can sometimes be exciting ("He will be able to go back to work—we need the money"), and it can also sometimes be concerning ("She may not need me as much now that the anxiety is improving"). Change will be gradual, and you both will have plenty of time to adjust.

- **Listen to what your loved one needs from you.** Most of us want to help our loved ones, especially when they are having a hard time. But sometimes, in an effort to be supportive, you may wind up doing things that only make it easier for your loved one to engage in anxiety-related behaviors. When your loved one is ready for you to stop doing things like providing reassurance, completing tasks that he finds too anxiety-provoking, or accommodating the anxiety in other ways, you need to be willing to stop. It may make things harder in the short-term, but it will pay off down the road.

- **Don't try to be your loved one's therapist.** It's not your job to solve her anxiety problem. In fact, your constant efforts to eliminate the anxiety can just make it worse. Emotional overinvolvement by family members can get in the way of a person's treatment.

- **Communicate.** Listen to your loved one and share your own feelings. Your input and support will be invaluable as your loved one takes some positive steps toward reclaiming his or her life. You may find that your relationship ends up stronger than ever with your help.

Other Ways to Involve Your Family

In addition to enlisting them as helpers, there are ways to involve family members in your program. Your family may be trying help you avoid the situations you fear because they want you to feel comfortable. If you're afraid to enter supermarkets, maybe your spouse does all grocery shopping. If you're afraid to get behind the wheel, perhaps your adult daughter does all the driving. If you're afraid of dogs and cats, your partner might be used to checking the area outside your house for dogs and cats before you leave home.

If your family members are trying to help you in these ways, they may have to be instructed to stop. Although they may have your best interests at heart, helping you avoid the things you fear may make it more difficult for you to overcome your anxiety. You may find it hard to give up this help—and may even create tension in the relationships by doing so—but it's an important step toward overcoming your anxiety. Of course, family members should be supportive and understanding, but there's a big difference between being supportive and enabling you to avoid the situations you fear.

Seeking Professional Help

There is evidence that self-help books like this one can be useful for treating certain anxiety problems even without the help of a professional therapist. Other people need a friend, a relative, or a therapist to check in on them from time to time. In fact, self-help treatments for anxiety are most effective when combined with occasional brief visits with a professional to check on progress and make sure that the treatment is on track. Others benefit most from seeing a professional and using self-help materials as a supplement to the therapy. In this section, we'll help you decide whether to seek professional help and how to select a professional who will provide the most help.

Deciding Whether to Seek Professional Help

First of all, don't feel stuck with any decision you make about whether to seek professional help. You may decide to begin this program without the help of a therapist, but you can always change your mind if it turns out that you need extra support or guidance. Here are three factors to consider as you decide whether to hire a professional.

The Severity of Your Anxiety

Generally, the more severe your anxiety problem, the more likely you are to benefit from therapy with a professional, as opposed to an exclusively self-help approach. If you have multiple anxiety problems or if they are very impairing or distressing, you may want to try working with a professional in addition to using this book.

The Way You Prefer to Get Things Done

If you usually prefer to work collaboratively, then working with a therapist may be a good option, in addition to using this book. A therapist can help keep you motivated, join you for practices, provide emotional support, and answer your questions along the way. On the other hand, if you like to work independently, are a self-starter, and are able to stick to a schedule without the support of others, then working on your own may be fine.

Medication Treatment

If you would like to start or continue medication as part of your treatment, you'll need the help of a prescribing professional. Far too many people "self-medicate" with drugs or alcohol. If this describes you, you may be well advised to talk to someone about pharmaceutical treatments.

How to Choose Professional Help

A first step in finding professional help is to decide what type of treatment you're seeking. Medication? Psychotherapy? A combination of the two? Some other approach? Next, consider the availability of various treatment options. In big cities, you may have the luxury of being able to choose among a large number of mental health practitioners who have experience in treating anxiety using a wide range of methods. You may even have one or more clinics in your city that specialize in treating anxiety disorders. On the other hand, you may live in a community where you have few choices. Regardless, knowing what your options are will help you make an informed decision.

Cost of treatment is a third consideration. If you have insurance or live someplace where mental health treatment is covered under national health insurance, make sure you know what your plan will cover. And don't forget to consider both the short-term and long-term costs of treatment. Although medication treatments may cost less in the short term, over the long term the cost can add up, whereas cognitive-behavioral therapy (CBT) is often less expensive over time. This is because medication use generally continues for a much longer period (several years) compared to cognitive-behavioral treatments, which typically last only a few months.

Keep in mind that some universities have sliding-scale clinics in their psychology departments where you can receive CBT from a trainee who is supervised by a licensed psychologist. There may also be opportunities to receive treatment in the context of a research study for a reduced fee or even at no charge.

Regardless of which approach you choose, find a professional who is experienced in treating anxiety disorders using methods that have been shown to be effective. In mental health care, not all therapies are equivalent. Many practitioners use methods that are not necessarily proven to be helpful for particular problems. Be informed about what methods are most likely to be useful. It's also a good idea to interview your prospective therapist to make sure that he or she can offer what you're looking for. Examples of questions to ask include:

- What experience do you have in treating anxiety and related disorders? (Look for some-one with experience.)

- What are your professional credentials? (Look for someone who has formal credentials, such as a psychologist, psychiatrist, social worker, or other mental health professional.)

- What sorts of approaches do you use to treat anxiety and related disorders? (Look for someone who uses exposure-based strategies, behavior therapy, cognitive therapy, CBT, medications, or combinations of these approaches.)

There are a number of ways to find an experienced therapist. You can contact a reputable professional association that provides referrals to members who specialize in treating anxiety and related disorders. There are also organizations that specialize in particular types of anxiety problems. See the Resources at the back of this book for listings of organizations that can help you identify professionals near you that are available to help. Other ways of finding professional help include speaking with your family doctor, visiting a local mental health clinic (especially one that specializes in anxiety disorders, if one is available in your community), and talking to people you know (health care professionals, friends, coworkers, family members) who might be aware of available options. Some communities publish guides to accessing local mental health services, including lists of practitioners in the area. There may also be information about services in your community on the Internet.

Finally, a number of programs in the United States and elsewhere offer intensive treatments for anxiety problems (several of the referral sources listed in the Resources can help you find intensive treatment programs). These programs typically occur over a short period (for example, 3 weeks) and are offered either on an inpatient basis or as day treatment (with daily outpatient appointments). Because these intensive programs last only a few weeks, they are often a convenient option for people who are willing to travel to get help.

Make sure you find a therapist with whom you feel comfortable working—someone you trust and with whom you can share personal information. If you find you're not happy with your therapist after a few sessions, consider finding another one.

If you're thinking about trying medications, you will need to see a professional who can prescribe. This will often be a physician (typically a family doctor or psychiatrist). Nurse practitioners can also prescribe medications; in a small number of jurisdictions (Iowa, Idaho, Illinois, New Mexico, Louisiana, Guam, and some United States government branches, such as the military) some psychologists are allowed to prescribe medications. A good place to start is with your primary care physician, who can discuss the medication options and either prescribe the medications or recommend someone who can. See Chapter 4 for a discussion of the advantages and disadvantages of medication treatments versus other types of treatment.

4

setting goals and planning your program

As you work through this chapter, you'll be setting goals. If you're dealing with several different anxiety problems, you'll need to decide which problems you want to work on first and which can wait. Strategies for choosing among various treatment approaches and for developing a comprehensive plan will be discussed.

Setting Goals

An important strategy for keeping your program on track is to set goals. Setting goals will help you select appropriate treatment methods and make it easier to determine whether treatment is working (that is, whether your goals are being met). Reminding yourself of your goals on a regular basis also keeps your motivation strong as you work to reduce your anxiety. At the end of this section, you will have an opportunity to record your goals for the program (see Form 4.1).

Goals should be:
- **Mostly specific**
- **Short, medium, and long term**

Specific versus Broad Goals

Although it's okay to have a few broader goals, most of your goals should be as specific as possible. This makes it easier for you to select particular treatment strategies to meet your goals and to assess whether you're getting closer to meeting them. Here are some examples to help you understand the difference between specific and broad goals.

Examples of Specific Goals

- To stop having unexpected panic attacks
- To sit in the same room as a dog without feeling anxious

- To make at least three new friends over the next year
- To apply for at least five new jobs over the next month
- To leave the house each day regardless of how anxious I feel
- To stop all compulsive washing
- To cut down the frequency of worrying about my children by at least 50%
- To sleep at least 7 hours through the night
- To drive from work to home with minimal anxiety

Examples of Broad Goals

- To be less anxious and worried
- To be more satisfied with my job
- To reduce the frequency of anxiety-provoking thoughts
- To be happy
- To feel calm
- To have better relationships

Short-Term versus Long-Term Goals

As you develop your list of goals, include examples for the short term, the medium term, and the long term. Short-term goals might include objectives that you would like to reach in the first month of your treatment; medium-term goals might include those targeted for the next few months; and longer-term goals might include those that you intend to fulfill over the next few years. Of course, you can develop goals that cover any time period you want, from a few minutes from now to the next 30 years. Below are some examples of short-term, medium-term, and long-term goals for Leigh, who suffers from obsessive–compulsive disorder, or OCD (specifically, she feels the need to check her work repeatedly), as well as anxiety in social situations, occasional unexpected panic attacks, and occasional bouts of moderate depression.

Leigh's Short-Term Goals (for the Next 4 Weeks)

- To reduce her compulsive checking (for example, locks, stoves) to less than 1 hour per day
- To spend at least 2 hours per day working on her anxiety problems
- To begin thinking less anxiously when in social situations

Leigh's Medium-Term Goals (for the Next 4 Months)

- To eliminate all compulsive checking
- To be able to leave home without experiencing an intense urge to check the locks and stoves more than once

Treatment Goals

Record your goals for treatment. Be as specific as possible.	
Period	**Goals**
Short-term (next 4 weeks)	• _____ • _____ • _____ • _____
Medium-term (next 4 months)	• _____ • _____ • _____ • _____
Long-term (for the next 2 years)	• _____ • _____ • _____ • _____

- To no longer experience panic attacks

- To feel less anxious in social situations such as parties, work meetings, meeting new people, and dating

- To look for a new job (to apply for at least five jobs per week until finding one)

Leigh's Long-Term Goals (for the Next 2 Years)

- To be in a long-term relationship

- To have a new job that she enjoys

- To maintain the gains she has made with respect to her social anxiety, OCD, and panic attacks

- To no longer feel depressed

What goals do you have for your future? Record them on Form 4.1.

Choosing among Treatment Strategies

Chapters 5 through 13 each describe specific strategies for dealing with anxiety (the Conclusion is about maintaining your gains after completing the program). Depending on the types of anxiety problems you have, some of these approaches may be more relevant than others. The box below and on the facing page lists the strategies taught in each of these chapters and the types of problems they are most suited for.

Choosing among the Various Strategies in This Program

What is it?	Who should use it?
Cognitive strategies (Chapter 5 to 7) involve changing unrealistic, anxiety-provoking thoughts into more balanced, realistic thoughts.	These strategies are potentially useful for all anxiety-based problems, although they are used less often with very focused fears and phobias (for example, animal phobias, blood phobias), where exposure is the treatment of choice.
Exposure to fear triggers (Chapter 8) involves confronting feared situations, objects, thoughts, memories, images, feelings, and sensations instead of avoiding them.	Exposure to fear triggers is important for anyone who fears or avoids particular external objects and situations, as well as internal experiences, such as thoughts and feelings. This chapter also discusses strategies for eliminating safety behaviors that contribute to anxiety. Chapter 8 provides an introduction to exposure and should be read before reading Chapters 9, 10, or 11, which focus on particular types of exposure.

What is it?	Who should use it?
Exposure to feared situations (Chapter 9) involves entering feared situations and confronting feared objects and activities.	These strategies are very important for anyone who fears and avoids objects, places, situations, or activities, such as animals, driving, social situations, being alone, touching contaminated objects, flying, and just about any other situation that you may fear. All the anxiety disorders are associated with some amount of situational fear. The more you have been avoiding encountering particular objects or situations, the more important it is to include exposure as part of your treatment.
Exposure to feared thoughts, memories, images, and urges (Chapter 10) involves repeatedly bringing on frightening thoughts, images, or impulses until they are no longer frightening.	These strategies are useful for people who are frightened by their own thoughts, memories, images, and urges or who worry that these experiences may be dangerous in some way. Examples include people who are afraid to allow themselves to remember a traumatic event, people who worry that they may lose control or go crazy if they allow themselves to experience an anxiety-provoking thought or image, people who worry that they may act on their unwanted impulses (often the case in OCD), and people with height phobias who worry they will be drawn to the edge of a high place and jump.
Exposure to feared feelings and sensations (Chapter 11) involves exercises (for example, spinning, overbreathing, aerobic exercise) designed to bring on feared sensations repeatedly until they are no longer frightening.	These strategies are useful for people who are afraid of experiencing certain physical feelings and sensations. Examples include people who are afraid of a racing heart, who fear the consequences of dizziness, or who worry about feeling breathless. Fear of physical symptoms may occur broadly (for example, a person who fears feeling dizzy whenever it happens) or only in certain situations (for example, a person who fears feeling dizzy only when driving or a person who feels breathless only when in enclosed places).
Relaxation techniques (Chapter 12) involve learning to relax the muscles of the body and breathe more slowly.	Relaxation-based strategies are most useful for people who experience significant generalized anxiety, worry, and stress in their lives. They are less useful for people whose fear is tied to specific situations, such as driving, spiders, or public speaking.
Mindfulness and acceptance-based strategies (Chapter 13) involve developing skills to accept anxiety feelings rather than fight them.	Mindfulness and acceptance-based strategies are becoming more accepted and studied as a treatment for anxiety generally and for some anxiety disorders. Evidence suggests that they may be useful for generalized anxiety, worry, and stress, and learning to accept feelings of anxiety (rather than fighting them) can be a useful approach when combined with exposure and cognitive strategies for other anxiety-related problems.
Living without anxiety (the Conclusion)	Regardless of which types of anxiety problems you experience, you should review the material in the Conclusion. Strategies for preventing relapse are important for staying well.

What's Worked in the Past and What Hasn't?

Have you had treatment for anxiety in the past? If so, think about what worked and what didn't. If a particular approach (for example, exposure, cognitive therapy, medication) was useful in the past, consider trying it again. If a particular approach was not effective in the past, try something else this time. But consider whether unsuccessful past treatments didn't work for a reason (for example, stopping a medication too soon, taking a medication at a lower-than-recommended dosage, not completing homework, and so on). If you think you may be able to do things differently this time around, it may be worth trying a past treatment again, even if it was not totally successful.

Developing a Comprehensive Plan

Which strategies will best help me overcome my anxiety?

Your plan should include strategies for dealing with the most important aspects of your anxiety. Strategies are organized in this book in the same order that you should introduce them into your own therapy. The specific techniques you use will depend on your unique anxiety profile.

Start with the cognitive strategies described in Chapters 5–7. Virtually everyone with anxiety problems will benefit from these strategies. After a couple of weeks of practice in identifying and challenging your assumptions, introduce exposure-based strategies, as described in Chapters 8–11. Use situational exposure (Chapter 9) to deal with fear and avoidance of external objects and situations. Use cognitive or imaginal exposure (Chapter 10) if you're frightened of your thoughts, memories, images, or impulses. Use symptom exposure (Chapter 11) if you're afraid of the bodily sensations associated with anxiety.

Depending on the focus of your fear, you may not need all three types of exposure. And once you introduce exposure into your therapy, you should continue to use the cognitive strategies as well. In addition, while working on your exposure practices, it's important to begin to reduce or eliminate safety behaviors, as described in Chapter 8.

Strategies based on relaxation (Chapter 12) and mindfulness (Chapter 13) can be integrated into your therapy either after you've been practicing exposure or earlier in the treatment. For most anxiety problems, it won't be necessary to use the relaxation- and mindfulness-based strategies at all—exposure and cognitive strategies are quite powerful on their own. But problems such as generalized anxiety, worry, and stress management may respond well to the techniques described in Chapters 12 and 13, either as an alternative to the other approaches discussed in this book or as part of a comprehensive plan.

As you work through the strategies described in this book, keep in mind the issues discussed in Chapter 3 on how to deal with obstacles. As you encounter obstacles or challenges along the way, refer back to it. Finally, your program should end with attention to strategies for preventing relapse and return of symptoms, as described in the Conclusion.

Based on what you've read in this chapter, complete Form 4.2. Read each problem area in the left column and put a check in the middle column if it's a problem for you. This will

FORM 4.2

Selecting Relevant Treatment Components

Do I have this problem?	Check here	Strategies I should try
I experience anxious thoughts, worries, and predictions that make me feel unsafe		• Cognitive strategies—Chapters 5 to 7 • Mindfulness- and acceptance-based strategies—Chapter 13
I have fears that are triggered by objects, places, situations, or activities		• Confronting your fears—Chapter 8 • Exposure to feared situations—Chapter 9
I have fears that are triggered by thoughts, memories, images, urges, or uncertainty		• Confronting your fears—Chapter 8 • Exposure to feared thoughts, memories, images, and urges—Chapter 10
I have fears that are triggered by certain feelings or sensations in my body		• Confronting your fears—Chapter 8 • Exposure to feared feelings and sensations—Chapter 11
I carry a lot of stress and tension in my body		• Learning to relax—Chapter 12 • Mindfulness- and acceptance-based strategies—Chapter 13
I don't want my anxiety to come back		• Preventing your anxiety from returning—Conclusion

From *The Anti-Anxiety Program, Second Edition*, by Peter J. Norton and Martin M. Antony. Copyright © 2021 The Guilford Press. Purchasers of this book can photocopy and/or download additional copies of this material (see the box at the end of the Contents).

highlight which techniques and chapters we recommend you focus most on. Of course, there is nothing wrong with reading the other chapters; after reading them you may realize that they applied to you more than you thought. You can always revise your responses as you learn more about these strategies throughout this workbook. Take a look at Valerie's sample completed form as well.

A couple of things to notice. First, the Conclusion (preventing your anxiety from returning) should be checked by everyone. It would be silly to go through all of the work in this program and not take steps to make sure the improvements will stick with you. Everyone should conclude the program with this chapter. Second, all of the "I have fears that are triggered by . . ." problem areas suggest that you should read and work through Chapter 8 (on confronting your fears). This is an important general chapter that should be read and completed before you start Chapters 9, 10, or 11. In other words, it should be read by everyone undertaking the program.

The sample completed forms for Valerie, Jacob, Bindi, and Jacqui provide examples of the programs developed by the four people you read about in the Introduction. If any of them seemed particularly similar to you, pay special attention to their plan!

SAMPLE COMPLETED FORM 4.2 *(Valerie)*

Selecting Relevant Treatment Components

Do I have this problem?	Check here	Strategies I should try
I experience anxious thoughts, worries, and predictions that make me feel unsafe	✓	• Cognitive strategies—Chapters 5 to 7 • Mindfulness- and acceptance-based strategies—Chapter 13
I have fears that are triggered by objects, places, situations, or activities		• Confronting your fears—Chapter 8 • Exposure to feared situations—Chapter 9
I have fears that are triggered by thoughts, memories, images, urges, or uncertainty	✓	• Confronting your fears—Chapter 8 • Exposure to feared thoughts, memories, images, and urges—Chapter 10
I have fears that are triggered by certain feelings or sensations in my body		• Confronting your fears—Chapter 8 • Exposure to feared feelings and sensations—Chapter 11
I carry a lot of stress and tension in my body	✓	• Learning to relax—Chapter 12 • Mindfulness- and acceptance-based strategies—Chapter 13
I don't want my anxiety to come back	✓	• Preventing your anxiety from returning—Conclusion

SAMPLE COMPLETED FORM 4.2 *(Jacob)*

Selecting Relevant Treatment Components

Do I have this problem?	Check here	Strategies I should try
I experience anxious thoughts, worries, and predictions that make me feel unsafe	X	• Cognitive strategies—Chapters 5 to 7 • Mindfulness- and acceptance-based strategies—Chapter 13
I have fears that are triggered by objects, places, situations, or activities		• Confronting your fears—Chapter 8 • Exposure to feared situations—Chapter 9
I have fears that are triggered by thoughts, memories, images, urges, or uncertainty	X	• Confronting your fears—Chapter 8 • Exposure to feared thoughts, memories, images, and urges—Chapter 10
I have fears that are triggered by certain feelings or sensations in my body	X X	• Confronting your fears—Chapter 8 • Exposure to feared feelings and sensations—Chapter 11
I carry a lot of stress and tension in my body		• Learning to relax—Chapter 12 • Mindfulness- and acceptance-based strategies—Chapter 13
I don't want my anxiety to come back	X	• Preventing your anxiety from returning—Conclusion

Selecting Relevant Treatment Components

Do I have this problem?	Check here	Strategies I should try
I experience anxious thoughts, worries, and predictions that make me feel unsafe	✓	• Cognitive strategies—Chapters 5 to 7 • Mindfulness- and acceptance-based strategies—Chapter 13
I have fears that are triggered by objects, places, situations, or activities	✓	• Confronting your fears—Chapter 8 • Exposure to feared situations—Chapter 9
I have fears that are triggered by thoughts, memories, images, urges, or uncertainty	✓	• Confronting your fears—Chapter 8 • Exposure to feared thoughts, memories, images, and urges—Chapter 10
I have fears that are triggered by certain feelings or sensations in my body		• Confronting your fears—Chapter 8 • Exposure to feared feelings and sensations—Chapter 11
I carry a lot of stress and tension in my body		• Learning to relax—Chapter 12 • Mindfulness- and acceptance-based strategies—Chapter 13
I don't want my anxiety to come back	✓	• Preventing your anxiety from returning—Conclusion

Selecting Relevant Treatment Components

Do I have this problem?	Check here	Strategies I should try
I experience anxious thoughts, worries, and predictions that make me feel unsafe	Χ	• Cognitive strategies—Chapters 5 to 7 • Mindfulness- and acceptance-based strategies—Chapter 13
I have fears that are triggered by objects, places, situations, or activities	Χ	• Confronting your fears—Chapter 8 • Exposure to feared situations—Chapter 9
I have fears that are triggered by thoughts, memories, images, urges, or uncertainty	Χ	• Confronting your fears—Chapter 8 • Exposure to feared thoughts, memories, images, and urges—Chapter 10
I have fears that are triggered by certain feelings or sensations in my body		• Confronting your fears—Chapter 8 • Exposure to feared feelings and sensations—Chapter 11
I carry a lot of stress and tension in my body		• Learning to relax—Chapter 12 • Mindfulness- and acceptance-based strategies—Chapter 13
I don't want my anxiety to come back	Χ	• Preventing your anxiety from returning—Conclusion

Other Strategies to Consider

The rest of this chapter discusses other strategies for overcoming anxiety problems that some people choose to try, either in combination with or instead of this program. These include medications, complementary and alternative treatments, and lifestyle approaches. They aren't core parts of the program, but many people are already doing some of these things or considering adding them to their program. The information should help you make informed decisions about how best to proceed for yourself.

Medications for Anxiety Disorders

For most people, medications should be considered only if the other strategies are not effective on their own. That's because medication treatments for anxiety disorders are generally associated with higher rates of relapse following the end of treatment than are cognitive and behavioral approaches. Nevertheless, if cognitive behavioral therapy (CBT) is unavailable in your community or is not effective for your symptoms, or if you have a strong preference for medications, drug treatments are likely to be effective. They can be used right from the start of treatment or added later, after CBT has been given a chance to work.

While all medication decisions should be made in consultation with a prescribing health professional (for example, a physician or nurse practitioner), here is some general information about different classes of medications used to treat anxiety and related disorders (see the box below and on the facing page).

Medications Shown to Be Effective for Treating Anxiety and Related Disorders

SSRIs (selective serotonin reuptake inhibitors)

- escitalopram (Lexapro/Cipralex)
- fluoxetine (Prozac)
- fluvoxamine (Luvox)
- paroxetine (Paxil)
- paroxetine CR (Paxil CR)
- sertraline (Zoloft)

SNRIs (selective serotonin and norepinephrine reuptake inhibitors)

- venlafaxine XR (Effexor XR)
- duloxetine (Cymbalta)

Tricyclic Antidepressants

- clomipramine (Anafranil)
- imipramine (Tofranil)

Benzodiazepines

- alprazolam (Xanax)
- clonazepam (Klonopin/Rivotril)
- diazepam (Valium)
- lorazepam (Ativan)

Other Medications

- pregabalin (Lyrica), an anticonvulsant with good evidence for treating GAD
- buspirone (Buspar) for GAD
- adjunctive antipsychotics such as risperidone (Risperdal) for treatment-resistant disorders, especially OCD

Note: These medication names are those used in the United States and Canada. Names of medications may vary in other countries.

Selective Serotonin Reuptake Inhibitors

For many anxiety-related disorders, selective serotonin reuptake inhibitors (SSRIs) are often the first choice among medications. SSRIs act on a neurochemical in the brain called serotonin, by preventing neurons from reabsorbing unused serotonin. This effectively increases the amount of serotonin in the brain. It is unclear how this helps alleviate anxiety, however. SSRIs are classified as antidepressants, but they also work for anxiety and a variety of other problems, typically showing effects (compared to placebo) within a few weeks. Although different SSRIs are approved by the United States Food and Drug Administration (FDA) for certain anxiety disorders, there is enough evidence to suggest that they're about equally effective in treating most anxiety-related disorders, including panic disorder, social anxiety disorder, OCD, posttraumatic stress disorder (PTSD), and generalized anxiety disorder (GAD). The main exception is specific phobias, for which there is little research supporting SSRIs (or any other medications). The most common side effects from taking SSRIs include sexual dysfunction, weight gain, and sleepiness, though other common side effects include nausea, diarrhea, headache, sweating, anxiety, tremor, dry mouth, palpitations, chest pain, dizziness, twitching, constipation, increased appetite, fatigue, thirst, and insomnia. Fortunately, most people experience few (if any) of these symptoms, and they're usually mild in nature. Generally, SSRIs are relatively easy to discontinue. An exception is paroxetine (Paxil), which should be discontinued slowly. If paroxetine is stopped suddenly, or if doses are missed even for a few days, an individual is likely to experience symptoms such as sleep problems, anxiety, nausea, diarrhea, dry mouth, vomiting, sweating, and other uncomfortable feelings.

Selective Serotonin and Norepinephrine Reuptake Inhibitors

Selective serotonin and norepinephrine reuptake inhibitors (SNRIs) act on two different neu-rotransmitter systems in the brain: serotonin and norepinephrine. As with SSRIs, it is unclear how or why this can help alleviate anxiety disorders. Like SSRIs, SNRIs typically take a few weeks to kick in once an adequate dose is reached. Common side effects include constipa-tion, loss of appetite, nausea, dry mouth, dizziness, insomnia, nervousness, sexual dysfunction, sleepiness, sweating, and weakness, among others. SNRIs, particularly venlafaxine, should be stopped gradually after prolonged use to avoid uncomfortable discontinuation symptoms.

Tricyclic Antidepressants

This class of medications first appeared in the 1950s, with the introduction of a drug called imipramine. Although there are more than a dozen tricyclic antidepressants, only two, clomip-ramine and imipramine, have been studied extensively for treating anxiety and related disorders (clomipramine for OCD and imipramine for panic disorder). Side effects differ among the vari-ous tricyclic antidepressants but tend to include dry mouth, constipation, blurred vision, seda-tion, sexual dysfunction, sweating, and dizziness. Side effects and potential health risks tend to be more problematic with tricyclic antidepressants than with the newer classes of antidepres-sants like SSRIs or SNRIs, so they're prescribed less frequently than they used to be.

Benzodiazepines

Benzodiazepines are considered minor tranquilizers, and their main effect is to slow down the central nervous system. They are most often prescribed as treatments for anxiety, insomnia, seizures, muscle spasms, tension, or alcohol withdrawal. More than 15 benzodiazepines are available, though only four have been studied extensively for the treatment of anxiety disorders. Unlike antidepressants, benzodiazepines work quickly, often within a half hour. Therefore, they can be taken shortly before entering an anxiety-provoking situation. But many anxiety experts recommend taking a regular daily dose rather than taking these medications on an as-needed basis. As with other medications, different benzodiazepines have been approved for certain anxiety disorders. Common side effects of benzodiazepines include sleepiness, lightheadedness, confusion, dizziness, unsteadiness, depression, headache, insomnia, and nervousness. These drugs may also interfere with your ability to drive safely or to operate machinery. Benzodiaz-epines interact strongly with alcohol, so you shouldn't drink alcohol when taking these drugs. Older adults should use caution when taking benzodiazepines because higher dosages have been associated with an increased likelihood of falling.

One disadvantage of benzodiazepines is that they can be difficult to discontinue. Stopping these drugs abruptly can trigger intense anxiety, panic attacks, insomnia, and even seizures. Withdrawal symptoms are worse when they've been taken at higher dosages and for longer durations. It's extremely important to discontinue these medications very gradually, under the supervision of your doctor. Because of the difficulty of discontinuing them, these drugs are typically not the first choice for long-term treatment of anxiety-related problems.

Antipsychotic Medications

Antipsychotic drugs are used primarily to treat schizophrenia and related disorders, but they are also sometimes used to treat a range of other problems, including dementia, bipolar disorder, depression, and anxiety-related disorders. In the case of anxiety-related disorders, these drugs are most often used as adjunctive (or add-on) medications to enhance the effects of antidepressants, such as the SSRIs. Some of the antipsychotic medications that have been studied for anxiety include risperidone (Risperdal), haloperidol (Haldol), olanzapine (Zyprexa), quetiapine (Seroquel), aripiprazole (Abilify), and ziprasidone (Geodon). Although evidence is inconsistent for most anxiety problems, and none of these medications is approved by the FDA for treating anxiety-related disorders, the evidence supporting the use of risperidone for OCD is more consistent, with studies generally supporting the use of risperidone when added to an SSRI for individuals who don't respond to an SSRI alone. However, that doesn't mean that people with OCD should necessarily add risperidone to their SSRI. In fact, there is evidence that for people with OCD who have not responded to an SSRI alone, adding exposure-based strategies is more effective than adding risperidone. In addition, antipsychotic medications should be used sparingly in the treatment of anxiety-related disorders, given their side effects and the fact that many other treatment options are safer and easier to tolerate.

Other Medications

A number of other medications have been found to be useful for treating anxiety and related disorders. Certain anticonvulsants may be useful. For example, the use of pregabalin (Lyrica) has been supported in several controlled studies for the treatment of GAD and social anxiety disorder. In addition, Buspirone (Buspar) is an anxiolytic (though not a benzodiazepine) that has been found to be useful for GAD, but not other anxiety disorders. There are many other medications that have been studied as treatments for anxiety, though most require additional research before they can be recommended.

Herbal, Alternative, and Complementary Medicines for Anxiety Disorders

Alternative and complementary treatments are becoming increasingly popular in our society. In fact, a 2002 survey found that 62% of adults in the United States had used complementary and alternative therapies in the past year for a health concern, and another survey in 2012 found that half of college students had used an herbal product for anxiety in the past year. Treatments such as aromatherapy, Bach flower remedies, hypnotherapy, massage, nutrition, reflexology, reiki, and yoga have all been used to treat anxiety and stress. What does research tell us about the effectiveness and safety of such treatments? In most cases, there is very little or no good-quality research on these approaches for treating anxiety. In other cases, the existing research has numerous flaws (such as inappropriate or invalid measures of anxiety, inadequate numbers of participants, poorly described methods, poor controls for expectations by the participant or the investigator, or lack of placebo comparison). Only in a few cases are there well-conducted studies supporting these treatments.

Similarly, herbal remedies have been used for centuries by many different cultures to treat anxiety and other emotional difficulties. As we just mentioned, there are few serious studies of their effectiveness. Consumers should also be aware that quality control for herbal products can be uneven. In North America, for example, these substances are not well regulated, and the amount of the active ingredient in each capsule or pill may vary from what is printed on the bottle and from brand to brand. If these products do work (beyond possible placebo effects), they probably reduce anxiety by altering brain chemistry, which means they may have associated side effects, interactions, and withdrawal symptoms, just like any other medications. Therefore, they should be used with caution. If you are taking medications, inform your physician of any supplements or herbal treatments that you are using or considering trying.

> **Tell your physician about any herbal supplements you are using or considering taking.**

Lifestyle Interventions for Anxiety Disorders

Factors involved in our general health also affect anxiety and the ability to make the most of a program like the one in this book, so as you go through this program it's wise to know how to maximize your resources.

Diet and Nutrition

Scientists in England have shown that changes in diet and lifestyle can improve your anxiety at least as much as regular treatment from your physician. The researchers took almost 70 patients with panic disorder and randomly gave them either routine care from a general practitioner or a lifestyle treatment program delivered by an occupational therapist. Their results showed that both treatments led to about the same amount of improvement in anxiety, with some hints that improvement may have been slightly better in the lifestyle treatment on average.

Despite these findings bolstering your motivation and ability to work through this program, and other evidence that a well-balanced diet can have a positive impact on our sense of well-being, there is no consistent evidence supporting any specific anti-anxiety diet. In other words, we know of no specific food or vitamin supplement that will effectively reduce anxiety-related disorders. Be cautious about outrageous claims on the Internet or in the media about a new superfood or nutritional supplement. These claims are usually made without any basis or solid research backing them up. Most countries around the world, however, do offer useful dietary recommendations that can help you achieve balance in what you eat.

Social Life

For some people, particularly those with social anxiety or agoraphobia, anxiety can be a very isolating condition. You may fear being around others; sometimes it just feels better to stay home, where you feel safest. This may be the saddest and most ironic thing about having an anxiety disorder, because social support is one of the strongest protective barriers against psychological and emotional problems. Quite simply, having people you can talk to seems to protect against stress and emotional problems. If anxiety around other people is a problem for you, we strongly encourage you to make social activities a priority on your Exposure Plan (see Chapter 8). The only way to feel more comfortable around people is to practice being around others.

But what if you don't have many friends or opportunities to socialize? There are some helpful pointers for developing new social supports and reconnecting with old friends. First, as anybody who has moved to a new city can tell you, it can be hard to make new friends. It's becoming much rarer these days for neighbors to come over with a casserole or to have a complete stranger strike up a conversation with you at the coffee shop, especially in larger urban centers. New friends don't just show up when you need them. You have to actively seek them. Strong friendships usually grow out of shared interests and values. Occasionally you may come across two friends with very different interests, but this is rare. It can be very hard to maintain friendships when two people have very different interests. Shared interests may be a common love of cooking, playing sports, quilting, gardening, reading crime novels, singing, or anything else that can help forge a bond between two people.

Second, just like any relationship, friendships take time to develop. Occasionally you may hear of two people who became best friends almost instantly, but that's pretty rare. More commonly, friendships grow over time. An interesting way to think about friendships is to picture them as a pyramid. Your best or closest friends would be at the top of the pyramid, and casual acquaintances at the bottom. Notice how much larger the bottom of the pyramid is than the top. It's typical to have a lot of people we consider casual acquaintances, fewer people we consider friends, even fewer who are close friends, and fewer still who are our best friends.

In most cases, friends move up the pyramid one step at a time. Allow people you meet to start as acquaintances. As you get to know some of them better, you might start to consider them friends. Eventually some of them may become good friends. If you and the other person are lucky, that person may become one of your closest friends. This process should usually go one step at a time. Forcing someone up the pyramid too quickly can backfire.

Finally, sometimes people say that they used to have many friends, but when their anxiety problems flared up, the friendships started to dwindle away. This isn't uncommon. As anxiety starts to limit what you can do or where you feel safe going, it creates fewer and fewer opportunities to spend time with your friends. Maybe your friends accommodated your anxiety for a while, but eventually they found it hard always to have to plan around your fears. Maybe you felt ashamed about your anxiety and simply stopped calling old friends. Whatever the case, it's not too late to try to rebuild those friendships. Reconnecting has an advantage over meeting new friends. When trying to make friends with new people you meet, you might find that you don't have anything in common with them, you don't like them, or your views or beliefs are not well matched. But when rebuilding an old friendship, you already know that the two of you are compatible as friends. Keep in mind, however, that rebuilding friendships has some similarities to making new friends. You may find that old friends come back lower on your pyramid than they were before. Give the renewed friendship time to grow, just as you would with new friends.

Physical Exercise

Exercise is a powerful tool for reducing anxiety, as well as stress and depression. In fact, regular exercise for as little 30 minutes a day can have as big an impact on your anxiety as medications or therapy! Exercise is seldom prescribed as part of a treatment plan for anxiety, but it would be a good idea to add it yourself.

We don't know *how* exercise manages to reduce anxiety. It might be due to our brains releasing endorphins (the "happy" brain chemicals that our bodies produce naturally when exercising), changes in other brain chemicals, improvements in our self-image, or just a by-product of getting out and doing things instead of hiding indoors all day. Whatever the reason, exercise is a great way to reduce anxiety and stress.

Only your physician or an experienced personal trainer can help you decide what exercises would be best for you, given your age, weight, and fitness level. But remember that exercise and fitness aren't just about running marathons or lifting weights at the gym. Going for a brisk walk at the park for 30 minutes can be just as helpful. Healthy exercise programs can be designed for everyone, whether you're already fit or you have problems with excess weight or obesity, medical issues, or even a disability or problems with mobility.

And exercise does not need to be boring! Exercising through group activities is one way to make the process more fun, and it combines the benefits of exercise with the benefits of social activity. Sign up for an aerobics class, play on a recreational soccer team, or join a walking or running club. Find activities that you will enjoy. Needless to say, you'll be much more likely to stick with activities that you find fun than activities that bore you. You will be surprised at how beneficial it is for your physical and mental health.

Sleep and Anxiety

Does your anxiety interfere with the amount of sleep you're getting? Does it affect the quality of your sleep? If so, you're not alone. Up to two-thirds of people who seek treatment for an anxiety disorder also complain about insomnia. Worrying at night, panic attacks that wake you from your sleep, and even nightmares about traumatic events can all get in the way of getting a good night's sleep. But there is also strong research showing that poor sleep quality can make you even more vulnerable to experiencing anxiety and the negative effects of stress. Anxiety can cause impaired sleep, but impaired sleep can also cause anxiety.

As you work through this program and begin to overcome your anxiety problems, your sleep will likely begin to improve. But if not, speak with your physician or a sleep medicine specialist, who can help diagnose your sleep problems and prescribe highly effective treatments, including psychological treatments or medications, to help you sleep properly again. CBT is an effective treatment for insomnia. An excellent book describing how to use CBT strategies for insomnia in the context of anxiety and depression is *Quiet Your Mind and Get to Sleep* by Colleen Carney and Rachel Manber.

That completes your preparation for the program! Now let's try some proven strategies for freeing you from the clutches of anxiety.

PART II

THE CORE PROGRAM

Congratulations on making it through "The Prep." By now you should have a very detailed understanding of your anxiety and how it affects you, and you will have developed your own personalized plan for how best to work through the program. You are now ready to move on and start making positive changes in your life.

In Part II, you will learn about and engage in the most widely researched and effective strategies for overcoming anxiety problems. Part II starts with three chapters that are designed to help you identify and challenge the anxiety-related thoughts underlying your anxieties and fears. The first chapter (Chapter 5) is designed to help you identify and carefully examine your anxiety-related thoughts, beliefs, and assumptions. This chapter is critical, because before you can change something, you need to understand it. When we work through this program as part of therapy, we usually ask the person we are working with to practice the skills in Chapter 5 for about a week. That advice holds here; please practice the skills for at least one week before moving on.

Chapters 6 and 7 will teach you strategies for challenging and countering these anxiety-related thoughts to help you develop a more balanced view of the triggers that provoke your anxiety. We suggest reading Chapter 6 and then practicing the skills in it for at least a week before moving on to Chapter 7. The skills in Chapter 7 should also be practiced for a week.

Finally, Chapters 8, 9, 10, and 11 describe the most powerful component of the treatment. It can be tempting to jump ahead and start with this section, but we recommend waiting until you've learned the skills in Chapters 5, 6, and 7 first, as these earlier skills help to provide a foundation for what comes next. Chapter 8 will teach you about *exposure therapy*. Everyone should read this chapter carefully to develop a plan for which of the following chapters (9, 10, and 11) are likely to be most beneficial. Depending on your anxiety and fears, you may need to focus only on one of these chapters, or you may find that it's best to tackle two or all three of them. Chapter 8 will guide you through the process of figuring out what's right for you.

If there are objects, situations, or experiences that you avoid because of your anxiety, you should be prepared to spend a considerable amount of time practicing exposure therapy to get the most benefit possible. Typically, when we conduct therapy using this program, we aim for about 6 weeks of exposure therapy, although you may find that you want to spend more or less time than that, depending on your own anxiety and fears. We wish you all the success in the world in using the program to overcome your difficulties with anxiety!

5

identifying thinking patterns that contribute to anxiety

In this chapter you're going to start on your journey toward regaining control over your anxiety. We hope you'll be making some big changes in how you think, act, and feel. And this can sometimes be a bit unnerving, so we recommend doing a quick rehash of the cost–benefit analysis that you completed in Chapter 3 (see Form 3.1). Using Form 5.1, you can see whether your view of the pros and cons has changed since you read Chapter 3. Are you ready to push beyond those cons and embrace moving toward the pros? We hope so!

Anxiety-Related Thinking

Anxiety-related thoughts keep worry and fear alive. For example, if you think the plane is going to crash, you're going to feel on edge during the entire flight. The strategies in this chapter will help you become more aware of anxiety-provoking beliefs, assumptions, and predictions, which is useful for combating excessive worry, panic attacks, and anxiety triggered by all sorts of situations and experiences, including external fears (spiders, a stuck elevator, going to the mall, losing your job), as well as internal ones (a pounding heart, memories of a trauma, an inexplicable urge to hurt someone).

Almost all types of anxiety and fear are accompanied by thoughts of threat and danger. And there are certainly situations in which anxiety is entirely appropriate, as when a loved one is in the hospital with a serious illness. It's only when these emotions grow out of proportion to the actual danger or threat that they cause a problem, interfering with your social life, your business obligations, your ability to take care of your kids, and many other aspects of your life.

What kind of anxiety-related thoughts do I have?

FORM 5.1

Revisiting the Costs and Benefits of Using This Program

What are your long-term goals and desires? What would you like to do with your life in the next 1 to 3 years?

_____

_____

_____

_____

Now, thinking about your own anxiety and your own life, record the costs and benefits of (1) working through this program and (2) not working through this program.

Working through the program (0–100 importance)		Not working through the program (–100–0 importance)	
Pros _____ (____)		Pros _____ (____)	
_____ (____)		_____ (____)	
_____ (____)		_____ (____)	
_____ (____)		_____ (____)	
Cons _____ (____)		Cons _____ (____)	
_____ (____)		_____ (____)	
_____ (____)		_____ (____)	
_____ (____)		_____ (____)	

The Relationship between Thoughts and Feelings

Sita was running about 30 minutes late for a routine checkup at her family doctor's office. She had left home with enough time to get to the appointment, but traffic was backed up because of an accident. Sita had left her cell phone at home, so she had no way to reach the doctor's office to let them know. What emotions do you think Sita might have been experiencing as she sat in traffic?

There's no one right answer. Different people respond to identical situations in different ways, and those responses are translated into different emotions. Our beliefs, predictions, assumptions, and thoughts all influence how we feel from moment to moment. So what Sita feels as she sits in traffic is influenced by how she interprets the situation. Here are some examples of thoughts that might trigger various emotions for her:

"I'm going to be late and my doctor will be very angry." → **Anxiety**

"Those idiots should pull over so we can all get by!!!" → **Anger**

"I should have anticipated this delay. I can't do anything right!" → **Sadness**

"I was dreading this appointment—it's great to have an excuse to miss it!" → **Relief**

"This is not a big deal. I can just rebook the appointment if my doctor can't see me." → **Calmness**

Note how each interpretation or prediction leads to a very different emotional state. Also notice that one of Sita's predictions is that her doctor will be angry. But that's just one of many possible reactions that her doctor might have. What emotions do you think Sita's doctor might experience while waiting for Sita to arrive? Well, just as Sita's emotions are determined by her thoughts, her doctor's emotional response would likely be influenced by thoughts about Sita's delay. Here are some examples of emotions that Sita's doctor might experience, and the thoughts that might have led to each of these emotions:

> **Our *interpretation* of events dictates our emotional response.**

"I wonder if Sita is hurt or in some sort of trouble. She never misses an appointment!" → **Anxiety**

"Where the heck is she? This is costing me money!" → **Anger**

"Maybe Sita stood me up because she knows I'm not a very good doctor." → **Sadness**

"I'm running so far behind schedule today. With Sita not showing up, I may have a chance to catch up!" → **Relief**

"I'm sure Sita is late for a good reason. I'll just book her for another visit." → **Calmness**

Notice again how particular emotions are associated with particular types of thoughts. *Anxiety* is associated with interpretations involving themes of threat and danger. *Anger* can also occur when we view a situation as threatening (for example, if someone hurts our feelings), but anger and frustration can be triggered as well when we are prevented from reaching a goal (for example, sitting in bad traffic or being stuck on the runway and missing our flight connection). Feelings of *sadness* and depression often occur when we have experienced some sort of loss (for example, a demotion on the job, the breakup of a relationship) or when we experience thoughts involving themes of hopelessness (for example, "I will never find a partner"). Positive feelings of *relief* occur when a potential threat or danger is removed (for example, after finding out that a loved one has returned safely from a war zone), and general feelings of *calmness* occur in response to neutral or pleasant thoughts.

Pay attention to the relationship between your thoughts and your feelings. When you learn to change your anxiety-related thinking, you'll reduce your levels of anxiety and fear.

The Role of Unconscious Thoughts

At this point, you may be thinking, "Sometimes I get anxious and I don't really know why." There's no question that the interpretations that trigger anxiety and fear can occur outside of our awareness. In fact, the parts of the brain that process fear (located in an area known as the limbic system) are quite primitive. So although anxiety-provoking thoughts can trigger anxiety and fear, these emotions can also occur in response to unconscious appraisals of threat and danger. Even though you may experience anxiety or fear without understanding what triggered it, you can assume that in most cases your brain is interpreting your experiences as dangerous in some way. After all, fear and anxiety are the body's natural responses to some sort of perceived threat.

There are lots of examples of how we process information unconsciously. In his best-selling book *Blink,* Malcolm Gladwell provides a fascinating review of research demonstrating that quick, intuitive thinking—the kind that occurs in the "blink of an eye" (that is, unconscious information processing)—is very important in the process of making decisions, particularly in situations and during activities that are overlearned and very familiar to us.

For example, an experienced driver can safely negotiate traffic even while consciously thinking about things other than the road. Similarly, if a bear were to jump out in front of you while you were hiking in the woods, you would need to make a split-second decision about the best way to protect yourself—there would be no time for conscious thought. Conscious thought occurs much more slowly than the quick sorts of decisions we can make outside of our awareness. The sort of information processing that takes place in the limbic system allows your body to react very quickly so you can deal with situations immediately, long before conscious thought has a chance to kick in.

Such quick thinking is helpful in emergency situations. With any luck, you would use it to escape the bear. Intuition, unconscious decision making, and other forms of thinking outside of awareness can also get us into trouble, however. When you've experienced a particular anxiety problem for a long time, it may become second nature to appraise even safe situations as dangerous. These evaluations may occur outside of awareness, and you may then be afraid when there's no realistic threat.

It is just this sort of response that this chapter will help you change. The strategies in this chapter are designed to help you become more aware of your anxiety-related thoughts, beliefs, and interpretations. Becoming aware of your anxiety-related thinking is essential before moving on to the next two chapters, which provide strategies to consider new ways of understanding the situations you fear, select more realistic and balanced interpretations and predictions when possible, and test out the accuracy or truthfulness of your patterns of anxiety-related thinking.

The Role of Biased Attention and Memory

If our anxiety stems from negative thinking, why doesn't anxiety naturally decrease over time as we encounter the situations we fear and see that our anxiety-provoking assumptions don't come to pass? One reason is that we often avoid the situations and experiences we fear, so we never have a chance to learn that we needn't fear them. (We'll return to this issue in Chapter 8.) Another reason is that we often *ignore* information that doesn't fit with our views in favor of information that does. In fact, we tend to seek out information that is consistent with our expectations and beliefs. Check out "The Awareness Test" (*www.youtube.com/watch?v=Ahg6qcgoay4*). It's a great demonstration of how if you're looking for something, you'll find it, and if you are not looking for something you are likely to miss it.

Not only do we seek out and pay close *attention* to information that is consistent with our views, but we're also more likely to *remember* such information. In other words, what we see in the world and what we remember about it are not necessarily completely consistent with reality. Rather, our experiences are biased: they're influenced by our emotions and our expectations. If you're feeling sad, for example, you may dwell on sad things that have happened in your life (such as the loss of a relationship or a job) and interpret current situations more negatively. Similarly, if you're angry at your best friend, you may be more likely to interpret her late arrival for dinner as a sign of disrespect than you would at a time when you had kindly thoughts toward your friend.

The same holds true for anxiety. People who are anxious are more likely to pay attention to (and remember) information that is consistent with their anxiety-provoking beliefs than information that disconfirms these beliefs. Think about it:

- If you fear spiders, you'll be the first to spot a spider in a room (perhaps because you are unconsciously "looking" for spiders).

- When you fear flying, you may remember every detail concerning a plane crash reported in the news years earlier but pay little attention to the millions of planes that take off and land safely each year.

- People with panic attacks who anxiously anticipate a racing heart often scan their bodies for unusual heart sensations. Research has shown that they can also count their heartbeats more accurately than people who are not afraid of a racing heart.

For the next few days or weeks, practice identifying your anxiety-related thoughts whenever something triggers your anxiety. Use the top part of Form 5.2 to record your thoughts. (You can make extra copies of this form to record different incidences of anxiety or download and print additional copies; see the end of the Contents for information.) This may seem silly ("I know what I'm thinking!"), but it is part of a larger process. This first step is designed to help you *think about your thinking*. Identify the thought and then examine it. What are you really thinking? Why are you thinking it? And, as we'll discuss in the next section, what kind of anxiety-related thought is it? Describe the situation or trigger that made you anxious and then record three of the thoughts that came up about the situation or trigger.

Types of Anxiety-Related Thinking

Anxiety-provoking thoughts usually occur in the form of a prediction that something bad will occur (though they take other forms too). In this section we'll review thoughts and experiences

FORM 5.2

Practice Identifying Anxiety-Related Thinking

Describe the trigger that made you anxious or fearful:

_____

_____

List the anxiety-related thoughts you experienced:

1. _____

2. _____

3. _____

Pick the strongest of these anxiety-related thoughts and identify what type(s) of thought it is and why it fits under that type:

_____

☐ Probability overestimation   Why? _____

☐ Catastrophizing   Why? _____

☐ Rigid rules   Why? _____

☐ Anxiety-provoking assumptions   Why? _____

☐ Negative core beliefs   Why? _____

☐ Anxiety-provoking impulses   Why? _____

☐ Anxiety-provoking imagery   Why? _____

From *The Anti-Anxiety Program, Second Edition*, by Peter J. Norton and Martin M. Antony. Copyright © 2021 The Guilford Press. Purchasers of this book can photocopy and/or download additional copies of this material (see the box at the end of the Contents).

that can contribute to your anxiety. You'll see that these experiences are not completely distinct from one another—they overlap a bit. Understanding these types of anxiety-related thoughts will be particularly valuable as you use the strategies in the next chapters to change your own anxiety-provoking thoughts.

Probability Overestimation

Do you often assume that something bad is going to happen in certain situations you

Anxiety-Related Thinking
- Probability overestimation
- Catastrophizing
- Rigid rules
- Anxiety-provoking assumptions
- Negative core beliefs
- Anxiety-provoking impulses
- Anxiety-provoking imagery

fear, even though you've discovered over and over again that it doesn't? For example, someone who has a fear of flying may assume that the risk of the plane crashing is high. Overestimating the chances of something bad happening is very common among people with anxiety problems, and it's a phenomenon we call *probability overestimation*. This type of thinking may also include a superstitious component in which events that have no relationship to one another are assumed to be related (for example, "The plane is more likely to crash *if I'm on it*").

When we engage in probability overestimation, we fail to rely on statistical facts and rational thinking, relying instead on our emotions, gut feelings, anecdotes, or dramatic stories. A movie like *Jaws* or a dramatic television interview with a shark attack victim can have a much more powerful effect on our fear of swimming in the ocean than would statistics on shark attacks, which make it clear that deaths due to shark attacks are extremely rare. But one look at a shark attack victim and facts and figures fly out the window!

Examples of probability overestimation include statements such as these:

- "A racing heart is a sign that I'm probably having a heart attack."
- "Dizziness means that I'm probably going to faint."
- "I am going to get cancer."
- "If I park in the underground parking at work, I will get assaulted."
- "If I allow myself to think about my rape, I will go crazy or lose control."
- "I will make a fool of myself during my presentation."
- "Nobody would ever want to date me."
- "I will get into a car accident."
- "I will get sick if I touch things in public places."
- "I will run out of money and be broke forever."
- "My children will get hurt."
- "The elevator will get stuck when I am on it."

Of course, all these events are possible, but that certainly doesn't mean they're probable. One goal of this chapter is to help you start thinking about probabilities based on the *evidence* rather than on your assumptions.

Catastrophizing

Catastrophizing (also called *catastrophic thinking*) refers to the assumption that a particular outcome will be completely unmanageable if it happens. Rather than thinking about how we might cope with a particular negative event, when we catastrophize we think about how awful the imagined event would be and how we wouldn't be able to cope with it. Whereas probability overestimation refers to exaggerating the *likelihood* of an event, catastrophizing refers to exaggerating the *importance* of the event.

Here are some examples of thoughts that reflect catastrophic thinking:

- "It would be absolutely terrible to faint."
- "I won't be able to cope if I have to drive in bad traffic."
- "It would be a disaster if I were to be rejected by someone."
- "I couldn't manage if I were to panic on an airplane."
- "Getting stuck in an elevator is one of the worst things I can imagine."
- "If I lost my job, it would be a complete disaster."
- "It would ruin my day if my teenager were to get anything less than an A in school."
- "It would be terrible to be late for an appointment."

Each of these examples takes a situation that most people would find somewhat unpleasant or inconvenient and exaggerates its ill effect. The truth is that people manage situations like these all the time. Chances are that you can also manage certain situations that probably feel as though they would be unmanageable.

Rigid Rules

Rigid rules are inflexible beliefs we have about the way things *should* be (and often include words like *should* or *must*). Rules tend to be based on our own values, so it can be difficult to prove whether they're true or false. We can, however, examine whether particular rules are *helpful* (more on this later). The rules and expectations we have for how things should be often contribute to our anxiety.

Some examples of rules that may contribute to anxiety include:

- "I should never have bad thoughts about others."
- "I must hide my anxiety from others at all cost."
- "I should be able to make my anxiety go away."
- "I should never make mistakes at work."
- "I must get an A on my exam."
- "I can never be late."
- "Children should always listen to their parents."

You can probably see the interrelationships among the types of anxiety-provoking thoughts we have discussed so far. Someone with test anxiety, for instance, might mistakenly believe that he'll do poorly on an exam (probability overestimation), that it would be terrible to get less than an A on the exam (catastrophizing), and that it's always essential to do well on exams (rule). Now let's continue with some other forms of anxiety-related thinking.

Anxiety-Provoking Assumptions

Assumptions refer to our general beliefs about the way things are. Sometimes they're correct and sometimes they're not. If we suffer from anxiety, our assumptions often exaggerate the true level of risk or danger. These anxiety-provoking assumptions may lead us to make anxiety-provoking predictions, including probability overestimations and catastrophizing. If you assume that driving is very dangerous, for example, you may predict that you're likely to be in a car accident each time you get behind the wheel. Other examples of possibly false assumptions that can contribute to anxiety include:

- "Most large dogs are prone to attacking people."
- "There are always lots of drunk drivers on the road."
- "I'm not smart enough to do well on my exam."
- "It's possible to run out of air on an elevator."
- "People can get cancer from touching things that are contaminated."
- "People can tell when I'm anxious."
- "It's dangerous to feel dizzy."
- "Being anxious can lead people to go crazy or lose control."
- "Public bathrooms can transmit diseases."
- "Most people don't experience anxiety."

Negative Core Beliefs

A *core belief* is one that is deeply held and quite broad, as opposed to being focused on a specific situation. Core beliefs, which often begin in childhood, color the way we view most situations. When the content of core beliefs is negative, they can contribute to feelings of anxiety or depression, and other unpleasant emotions. For example, a person who has the core belief "I am incompetent" might constantly be anxious about looking stupid in front of others, about making mistakes, or about terrible things happening as a result of his incompetence (such as causing serious harm to others or never finding a life partner). Core beliefs can be about oneself, about other people, or about the world. Here are some examples:

- "The world is a dangerous place."
- "You can't trust anyone."
- "Things will always turn out badly."
- "I am a failure."
- "I am defective."
- "I am unlovable."

The general negative core belief doesn't necessarily have to be eradicated—often it's enough to work on the beliefs that arise in specific situations (for example, the car is going to crash) and ignore the question of whether more deeply held beliefs are in play. In other cases, spending some time working on your core beliefs can be helpful. This is particularly true for people who are depressed or who have experienced anxiety for a long time in a wide range of situations.

Anxiety-Provoking Impulses

Anxiety problems are sometimes associated with frightening impulses. People with obsessive–compulsive disorder (OCD) may worry that they'll do something terrible (for example, push someone into traffic, shout something embarrassing in public), even though they have no desire to do such things and have never acted on these impulses. This is very different from people who think about harming others and actually want to do so and who even act on the urges.

Phobias are also sometimes associated with irrational impulses that are scary, though not dangerous. For example, someone who fears driving may feel as though she might be "pulled" off the road or off a bridge by an overwhelming impulse. People with a fear of heights sometimes describe an urge to jump from a high place (this is different from someone who is suicidal and has thoughts about jumping).

Of course, our anxiety problems wouldn't make us do these things. For example, OCD doesn't lead people to act on their violent thoughts, and people with height phobias don't jump from high places. These impulses are actually just examples of probability overestimations. If we have these sorts of thoughts, we predict that we're going to act on our impulses, even though the chances of actually doing so are almost zero.

Anxiety-Provoking Imagery

Normally, when we use the term *thought,* we are referring to self-talk, or the things we say to ourselves. But our thoughts can also take place through imagery. For example, rather than *thinking,* "Wow, that was a beautiful painting in the museum," you might *imagine* the artwork in your mind's eye. This can happen with other senses as well. We can hum a song in our head or imagine another person's voice talking while we're daydreaming about a past conversation.

Some people describe their anxiety-provoking predictions in the form of images. For example, rather than *thinking about* a past trauma (like a serious accident at work), a person with posttraumatic stress disorder (PTSD) may have *vivid images* of the trauma. The images may be so vivid, in fact, that it feels as though the trauma is happening again (images of a past trauma that feel almost real are called *flashbacks*). For others, imagery is not so vivid but may still trigger anxiety. Someone who fears socializing, for example, may have images of going to a party and being laughed at or criticized. As you work through this chapter, practice identifying your anxiety-provoking imagery in addition to the other types of thoughts that occur when you're anxious.

Now that you have a better understanding of the types of anxious thinking, go back to Form 5.2 and identify if any (or many) of these types of thoughts seem to fit the anxiety-related thoughts that you recorded.

Jacqui's Anxiety-Related Thoughts

Jacqui is the woman we introduced earlier who has intrusive thoughts that she might somehow harm her newborn child. She was nervous about the idea of identifying her anxiety-provoking thoughts because she always worked so hard *not* to have those thoughts. But she decided to put her trust in the program and managed to fill out a few of the "Practice Identifying Anxiety-Related Thinking" forms. Sample Completed Form 5.2 shows one of her forms.

Troubleshooting

Although the strategies described in this chapter are effective tools for identifying the thinking patterns associated with anxiety and other emotions, obstacles sometimes arise along the way. Here is the most common problem that comes up, along with some possible solutions.

SAMPLE COMPLETED FORM 5.2 *(Jacqui)*

Practice Identifying Anxiety-Related Thinking

Describe the trigger that made you anxious or fearful: *Being in the nursery alone with my daughter while she was crying*
List the anxiety-related thoughts you experienced: 1. *She is crying because I have done something wrong*   2. *If she is hurt, it will be my fault*   3. *I am a bad mother and terrible person*
Pick the strongest of these anxiety-related thoughts and identify what type(s) of thought it is and why it fits under that type: *She is crying because I have done something wrong*   ☑ Probability overestimation   Why? *I don't actually know that anything is wrong*   ☐ Catastrophizing   Why? _____   ☐ Rigid rules   Why? _____   ☑ Anxiety-provoking assumptions   Why? *I'm assuming I must have done something wrong*   ☐ Negative core beliefs   Why? _____   ☐ Anxiety-provoking impulses   Why? _____   ☐ Anxiety-provoking imagery   Why? _____

Problem: "I can't figure out what my anxiety-related thoughts are."

Solution: First, if you're not aware of any specific anxiety-provoking thoughts (such as "If I have a panic attack, I will go crazy, lose control, or die"), try to identify whether there are some less specific thoughts that are influencing your fear (for example, "Something bad will happen, though I don't know what"; "I won't be able to cope with the anxiety feelings"; "the anxiety won't end").

Second, consider the possibility that instead of specific *thoughts*, perhaps anxiety-provoking *images* are contributing most to your anxiety. Are you aware of any such imagery?

Third, perhaps you're finding it difficult to identify thoughts because you're not actually anxious in this moment. Sometimes, triggering anxiety can help to make a person more aware of the anxiety-provoking thoughts. Try triggering your own anxiety by entering the situation you fear or imagining being in the situation. Then ask yourself again what sorts of anxiety-provoking predictions you're aware of.

If you still can't identify your anxiety-related thoughts, don't worry. The strategies you'll learn later in the book will be useful even if you can't identify these thoughts.

Problem: "I can't figure out what type of thinking my anxiety-related thoughts are" or "My anxiety-related thoughts seem to fit several types."

Solution: Many anxiety-related thoughts will have elements of multiple types of thinking. There may be, for example, elements of rigid rules and catastrophizing. Or they may not seem to fit neatly into any of them. Correctly classifying your thoughts is not essential to the program. What's important is that you can identify your anxiety-related thoughts and can see how they might not be perfectly accurate reflections of the real threat or danger.

Conclusion

Anxiety is often triggered by a tendency to assume that situations are more dangerous than they really are. Sometimes these anxiety-related thoughts are so quick and automatic that they occur outside our awareness. When we're anxious, we also tend to give greater weight to information that confirms our negative beliefs and to discount or ignore information that isn't consistent with these beliefs. This biased way of processing information helps keep our anxiety alive.

There are a number of types of anxiety-related thinking, including probability overestimations, catastrophic thinking, adhering to overly rigid rules, anxiety-provoking assumptions, negative core beliefs, anxiety-provoking impulses, and anxiety-provoking imagery. Once you are adept at identifying the thoughts that are driving your anxiety, it's time to move on to the next two chapters, which will teach you skills designed to counter and change the thinking patterns that contribute to your anxiety!

6

changing thinking patterns by evaluating the evidence

In Chapter 5, you learned about the importance of thoughts in driving your anxiety and practiced identifying and classifying the thought patterns that contribute to your anxiety. But before you can start working on changing your thoughts, you need to change the way you *think* about your thoughts. Most of us assume our beliefs are true. Of course, it's impossible for everyone's beliefs to be true (otherwise, we would all agree about everything!).

So let's assume for a moment that some of your beliefs are not true. For the purpose of this exercise, think about the beliefs that contribute to your anxiety as *guesses* or *hypotheses*. Question these beliefs and try to evaluate them the way a scientist or a detective would look for evidence and clues before settling on a conclusion.

Strategies for Changing Anxiety-Related Thoughts

When you get to the point where you can accept the idea that your beliefs are not facts, changing your anxiety-related thinking is a matter of three basic steps:

1. Becoming aware of your anxiety-provoking beliefs, assumptions, and predictions

2. Considering possible alternative beliefs, assumptions, and predictions

3. Evaluating the evidence regarding your anxiety-related beliefs, assumptions, and predictions, as well as the alternative beliefs you generated, and shifting toward a more flexible, balanced, and realistic way of understanding the situation

> 1. **Become aware**
> 2. **Consider alternatives**
> 3. **Evaluate evidence**

Becoming Aware of Your Anxiety-Related Beliefs, Assumptions, Rules, and Predictions

In Chapter 2 you began the process of identifying your anxiety-provoking thoughts and then expanded on that in Chapter 5. Go back to the lists you developed in Form 2.4 and Form 5.2 to refresh your memory. Feel free to add to the lists if you can think of any more.

Of course, making a list of your anxiety-provoking thoughts is just the first step. Now, whenever you experience feelings of anxiety or fear, ask yourself what you're thinking in that moment. Try to identify specific predictions that contribute to your discomfort and write them down on the Anxiety Thought Record (Form 6.1). This form should be completed whenever you experience particularly elevated anxiety (photocopy the form or download and print extra copies; see the end of the Contents for information on downloading). For now, just focus on the first three columns. When you experience anxiety, record the situation that triggered the anxiety (column 1), your anxiety-provoking thoughts and predictions (column 2), and your anxiety level (column 3). This form will also be used for challenging these thoughts. More details on how to use this form are provided later in this chapter.

This process of monitoring your thoughts should continue throughout the time you're working on overcoming your anxiety. The following are some examples of questions you can ask yourself to help you figure out what you're thinking. Questions like these are particularly useful for identifying probability overestimations, catastrophic thoughts, and anxiety-provoking impulses and images. They include general questions (particularly the first three), as well as those that are relevant to specific types of anxiety:

- "What am I afraid will happen?"

- "What do I predict will occur?"

- "What do I imagine will occur?"

- "What am I afraid will happen if I have a panic attack in a movie theater [unexpected panic attacks]?"

- "What will happen if I encounter a dog [dog phobia]?"

- "As I sit here worrying about my children, are there images that come to mind about what might happen to them [generalized anxiety and worry]?"

- "What will it mean about me if people don't like my presentation [public-speaking anxiety]?"

- "What will happen if I sit on a toilet seat in a public bathroom [fear of germs]?"

- "What do I think will happen to me if I drive on the high-way [fear of driving]?"

- "What will happen if I get a thought about hurting another person [obsessive–compulsive, aggressive impulses]?"

- "What do I think will occur if I think about my past trauma [posttraumatic stress]?"

My thoughts are just predictions.

Anxiety Thought Record

Situation	Anxiety-provoking thoughts and predictions	Anxiety before (0–100)	Alternative thoughts and predictions	Evidence and realistic conclusions	Anxiety after (0–100)

Identifying your assumptions can be challenging because, as we discussed, they often occur outside of awareness. The first step is recognizing that assumptions are *not* facts; they're just beliefs.

So how can you identify your own rigid rules or assumptions, discussed in Chapter 5? One way is to ask yourself, when you're feeling anxious or making negative predictions, whether there might be any underlying rigid rules or assumptions influencing your anxiety. For example, if you continually find yourself predicting that you're going to make a fool of yourself in front of others, is it possible that you believe others are always looking for flaws in your behavior (an assumption)? Or do you believe in the utmost importance of always making a good impression on others (a rule)? Or, if you're predicting that you are about to faint because you feel dizzy, perhaps you believe dizziness often leads to fainting (an assumption).

Core beliefs, discussed in Chapter 5, are perhaps the most difficult thoughts to make ourselves aware of. One strategy for identifying core beliefs is the downward-arrow technique. Essentially, this involves repeatedly asking questions to identify the deeper meaning of your anxiety-provoking predictions. Here's an example of how a therapist might use the downward-arrow technique with a patient named Brian, who suffers from social anxiety:

> BRIAN: I'm very worried about a meeting I have tomorrow. My boss is going to ask me to speak in front of the group.
>
> THERAPIST: What are you worried might happen?
>
> BRIAN: I'm afraid that I won't know what to say or that I may say something wrong.
>
> THERAPIST: Why would that be a problem?
>
> BRIAN: People will notice my mistakes.
>
> THERAPIST: So what?
>
> BRIAN: If they notice my mistakes, they'll think I'm stupid or incompetent.
>
> THERAPIST: Why would that be a problem?
>
> BRIAN: I guess that would mean that I really am incompetent.
>
> THERAPIST: Do you think you are incompetent?
>
> BRIAN: I guess part of me does think that.

In this example, Brian and his therapist identified a possible core belief that may contribute to his anxiety: "I am incompetent."

Considering Possible Alternative Beliefs, Assumptions, and Predictions

Another way to determine whether your beliefs are accurate is to take a broader perspective by considering other possible ways of thinking about the situation. For every anxiety-provoking thought, prediction, or interpretation, there are usually several possible alternative predictions and various different ways of understanding the situation. The box on pages 105–106 provides a number of examples.

Generating Alternative Beliefs

Anxiety-provoking situation and thoughts	Examples of alternative beliefs and interpretations
Situation: Your husband is 30 minutes late coming home from work, and he isn't answering his mobile phone. **Thought:** "He has been in a serious car accident."	"He stopped somewhere on the way home from work." "He left work late." "He is stuck in traffic." "He has been in a minor fender bender." "His phone is turned off." "The volume on his phone is turned down." "He is in a noisy place and can't hear the phone." "He is in an area with poor reception." "He left his phone at work or somewhere else." "The battery in his phone needs to be charged." "He is talking on the phone and can't take my call."
Situation: You have agreed to have lunch with some coworkers. **Thought:** "I will have nothing to say or I will say stupid things. They will think I'm stupid and boring!"	"They won't think I'm boring." "They won't think I'm stupid." "I will be able to think of intelligent things to say."
Situation: You are riding in an elevator. **Thought:** "The elevator will get stuck and I will suffocate."	"The elevator will not get stuck." "Even if the elevator gets stuck, I will not suffocate."
Situation: You are having a panic attack and feeling unreal and dizzy. **Thought:** "Dizziness means that I am about to go crazy or lose control."	"Dizziness can occur because I haven't eaten." "Dizziness can occur because of low blood pressure or standing up too quickly." "Dizziness can occur because of anxiety." "I may be experiencing dizziness simply because I am scanning my body looking for feelings of dizziness (I might not notice the feeling if I wasn't looking for it)." "People don't go crazy from dizziness." "People don't lose control from dizziness."
Situation: You are walking through the mall and someone walks toward you. **Thought:** "He is going to attack me or try to rob me."	"Perhaps he is just going to walk by me." "Perhaps he will ask me a question." "Perhaps he wants to tell me something." "Perhaps he is walking toward someone who is standing behind me."

Anxiety-provoking situation and thoughts	Examples of alternative beliefs and interpretations
Situation: An intrusive OCD thought about stabbing your wife pops into your head.	"Having a thought is not the same as acting on the thought."
	"I am not going to stab my wife."
Thought: "Thinking about stabbing my wife means that I'm likely to do it."	"Thinking about stabbing my wife doesn't increase the likelihood of doing it."

Recording Alternative Predictions

Use the fourth column of the Anxiety Thought Record (Form 6.1) to record alternative predictions.

Stepping into Somebody Else's Shoes

If you have difficulty coming up with alternative beliefs when you're feeling anxious, another strategy is to ask yourself how someone who doesn't have an anxiety problem might interpret the situation. You can even imagine someone in particular, like a close friend, partner, or relative (for example, "How would my best friend, who is comfortable in social situations, think about this party that I'm so anxious about attending?"). Chances are that this strategy will help you think of good alternatives. Remember that your natural tendency is to experience thoughts that are consistent with your anxiety. It will take conscious effort to generate different interpretations, beliefs, and predictions from the ones you've automatically had for years. But you will succeed if you stick with it.

Evaluating the Evidence and Selecting a Realistic Conclusion

Simply making a list of alternative beliefs and interpretations should help to decrease your anxiety because it will show you that your anxiety-related thoughts are just one way of thinking about the situations you fear. Next, we take the process a step further by evaluating the evidence for and against your negative thoughts, as well as for the alternative thoughts that you generated. This process is sometimes referred to as *challenging* your anxiety-related thinking. Record your evidence and realistic conclusions in the fifth column and then rerate your anxiety on a 0 (none) to 100 (worst imaginable) scale in the sixth column.

A number of different strategies can be used to challenge your anxiety-related thoughts, including educating yourself about the situations you fear and examining the evidence concerning the thoughts to evaluate the accuracy of your beliefs, predictions, and assumptions. Later in the chapter we discuss the most effective strategies for changing rigid rules and core beliefs.

Using the Anxiety Thought Record

As you work through the rest of this chapter, start to use the entire Anxiety Thought Record (Form 6.1) every time you feel anxious (or at least several times per week if your anxiety episodes are too numerous to record). There are six columns to complete:

1. Situation: Describe the situation that triggered your anxiety. This can be an object, activity, or experience (for example, a thought, memory, image, or physical feeling).

2. Anxiety-provoking thoughts and predictions: Record any anxiety-provoking thoughts or predictions that were on your mind. What were you afraid might happen?

3. Anxiety before (0–100): Using a scale ranging from zero (completely calm) to 100 (completely terrified), rate your anxiety level before you started to challenge your anxiety-related thoughts.

4. Alternative thoughts and predictions: Record a few alternative beliefs and predictions to counter the thoughts listed in column 2. What are some other possibilities?

5. Evidence and realistic conclusions: Using the strategies described in this chapter, record any evidence you can think of to counter your anxiety-provoking thoughts. Based on this evidence, write down a more flexible, balanced, and realistic conclusion or prediction.

6. Anxiety after (0–100): Using a scale ranging from zero (completely calm) to 100 (completely terrified), rate your anxiety level after you challenged your anxiety-related thoughts.

Education

You're not going to have an easy time figuring out whether your beliefs are true if there are important gaps in your knowledge about the situations you fear. One strategy for gathering evidence about the accuracy of your thoughts is to educate yourself. How you do this depends on the nature of the situations that make you anxious. The box below and on page 108 includes ways you can use education and information gathering to challenge anxiety-related thoughts for all kinds of anxiety issues. Sources of information can include other people (friends, relatives, experts), books, television, and the Internet.

Using Education to Challenge Anxiety-Related Thoughts

Issue	Strategies for gathering new information
"I'm concerned that others will think my presentation is boring."	Collect data at the end of your presentation and have attendees rate their satisfaction with various aspects of the presentation, including how interesting it was.
	Ask a few attendees whom you trust to provide honest feedback about your presentation.

Issue	Strategies for gathering new information
"I believe that snakes are dangerous."	Find out whether snakes in your area are in fact dangerous and how to distinguish between the dangerous ones and the harmless ones.
	Learn about the conditions under which snakes attack and how to tell whether a snake is likely to be aggressive.
	Find out what particular snake behaviors mean (for example, what does it mean when a snake sticks out its tongue?).
"I worry that my plane will crash, especially when I hear strange noises during a flight."	Seek out statistics on the frequency of plane crashes and the conditions under which crashes tend to occur.
	Learn about the meaning of various sounds that occur on planes.
"I worry that the elevator will get stuck and I will die of suffocation."	Seek out statistics (perhaps from a company that installs and repairs elevators) concerning how often elevators get stuck.
	Ask an expert how elevators are ventilated and whether it is possible to run out of air.
	Look for information about the frequency of elevator-related deaths.
"I'm convinced I'm going to be struck by lightning whenever there is a thunderstorm."	Learn more about thunderstorms, including how often they occur, how often people are struck by lightning, and how often people who are struck by lightning are severely injured or killed.
"I worry that my heart palpitations are a sign that I am having a heart attack."	Learn about the risks for heart disease and whether you have any of the most important risk factors.
	Arrange for a physical examination with your family doctor to rule out any medical problems (but don't do this over and over again—frequent and *repeated* reassurance seeking can maintain or even strengthen anxiety!).
	Learn about the signs and symptoms of heart disease.

Be sure to check multiple sources and be careful not to rely on sources that may be biased. Suppose you're trying to learn more about the risks of flying, for instance. Don't just check websites of the major airlines (which may underestimate the risks) or talk to others who fear flying (who may exaggerate the risks). Check out many neutral sources, such as the website of the National Safety Council, which provides statistics for death by various causes (*https://injuryfacts. nsc.org/all-injuries/preventable-death-overview/odds-of-dying*) and shows that the odds of dying in a plane crash are much less than from many other causes, including dying from a simple fall.

Balanced Thinking

Balanced thinking involves trying to shift your thinking by asking yourself questions such as "Do my thoughts make sense in light of all the information I have?" and "Are there other ways to look at this situation that make more sense based on the facts?" One example of a strategy for thinking more realistically is to examine your past experiences and use them to make more accurate predictions about the future. Consider the following discussion between Mike and his therapist:

MIKE: Every time I go into a public place like a restaurant or theater, I worry that I may have uncontrollable diarrhea and that I won't make it to the bathroom on time. It's easiest just to avoid these situations.

THERAPIST: Do you have that thought *every* time you're out in public?

MIKE: Well, not every time. Maybe about a third of the time.

THERAPIST: Of these times, how often have you actually had diarrhea?

MIKE: Not often. Maybe just two or three times. But the way my stomach rumbles, I sure feel like it's going to happen much more often than that. Besides, even two or three times is too many times to lose control of my bowels in public!

THERAPIST: Have you actually had diarrhea in public, or have you made it to a bathroom in time?

MIKE: Fortunately, I've always made it to the bathroom just in time. But I was lucky. Who knows what would have happened if I didn't have a bathroom nearby?

THERAPIST: Have you ever had the feeling that you needed a bathroom and couldn't get to one?

MIKE: Actually, that's happened a few times.

THERAPIST: What was the outcome?

MIKE: Eventually the feeling passed. I guess I didn't need the bathroom after all.

THERAPIST: So, of all the times you have been out in public, your feared consequence has never actually occurred. Even when you didn't have access to a bathroom, you survived without losing bowel control. What does that tell you about the next time you're in a public place?

MIKE: I guess the likelihood of having uncontrollable diarrhea is not as great as I think.

Notice how the therapist repeatedly asks Mike questions to help him come to a more realistic conclusion about his feared situation. We encourage you to ask yourself questions to challenge your own anxiety-related thinking. See the box on pages 110–112 for some suggestions.

Decatastrophizing

Decatastrophizing, just as it sounds, is a way to combat catastrophizing—as discussed in Chapter 5, that's when we exaggerate the importance of a possible event and assume that it will

Questioning Yourself to Challenge Anxiety-Related Beliefs

Anxiety-provoking belief	Examples of questions to ask yourself
"I worry that I'll make a fool of myself if I go to the party."	"What has my experience been in the past? Do I normally get feedback from others that I come across as foolish at parties?" "Don't most people say something foolish from time to time?" "Is it really so important that I come across perfectly? What are some of the benefits of allowing myself to make mistakes?" "So what if some people think I look foolish?" "What advice would I give to a close friend who was having this thought?"
"A spider will crawl on me, and I won't be able to cope."	"How often do I actually see spiders?" "Of those times, how often do they crawl on me?" "Am I generally able to cope okay in stressful situations?" "Based on my past experiences with spiders, what is the worst thing that will happen?" "How long will it take to get the spider off me? Will it really matter if a spider is on me for a few seconds or less?" "Other than feeling uncomfortable, are there any negative consequences? If not, can I handle feeling uncomfortable for a few seconds?"
"When I have a headache, I worry that it may be a brain tumor."	"How often have I had headaches in the past?" "How often do other people have headaches?" "What are some of the other triggers for my headaches?" "Have any of my past headaches been caused by a tumor?" "What are all the reasons people get headaches, other than tumors? How common are these other causes?" "Is it important to know what causes my headaches? Does the fact that I don't know the cause mean that it's a tumor?"
"I'm convinced that I will die in a car accident every time I get into a car."	"How often have I been in a car? Of those times, how often have I worried about getting into an accident? Of those times, how often have I actually been in an accident?" "What do I know about the percentage of accidents that are fatal (based on available statistics)?" "What does this tell me about the chances of dying in a car accident the next time I go for a drive?" "What are the factors that increase the risk of a car accident (for example, drinking, speeding, talking on the phone, following too closely, not paying attention)? Do I do any of those things?"

Anxiety-provoking belief	Examples of questions to ask yourself
"If I panic on a plane, I will drop dead of a heart attack."	"Is there any evidence that panic attacks cause heart attacks?"
	"Is there any evidence that a racing heart is dangerous? In fact, my heart races during exercise, and that's supposed to be good for the heart!"
	"What are all the reasons other than heart disease that hearts race (for example, arousal, exercise, anxiety, caffeine, paying attention to my heart rate)?"
	"What does my past experience tell me about the likelihood of dying during a panic attack? (I have panicked many times before and not died.)"
	"What are the risk factors for heart attack (for example, older age, smoker, overweight, high blood pressure, high cholesterol, family history of heart disease)? Do I have many of these?"
"I will lose control if I think about how I was abused as a child."	"What do I mean by 'lose control'?"
	"Have I ever actually lost control before?"
	"Does trying not to think about the abuse work, or does it lead me to think about it even more?"
"Others will notice my anxiety symptoms (especially my shaking) and will think I'm weak or strange."	"What else might people think if they notice my shaking (for example, they might think I'm cold)?"
	"Are there things other than 'I'm weak or strange' that people might think about me if they notice I am anxious?"
	"Does it really matter if some people think I am anxious (after all, I sometimes notice other people's anxiety, and they don't seem to suffer any negative consequences as a result)?"
	"Do I have the right to look anxious sometimes?"
	"Do people really notice every detail about others?" (If you are not sure, check out this video, called *The Door Study*, at *www.youtube.com/watch?v=FWSxSQsspiQ&t=13s.*)
"If I don't worry about my children, that means I'm a bad mother."	"Do children with worried mothers generally grow up healthier?"
	"Are there any negative consequences for me or my children of worrying about them too much?"
	"What would happen if I worried about my children even a bit less often?"
	"What advice would I give to a close friend who was having this thought?"
"It's important for everyone to like me."	"What would happen if someone didn't like me (for example, a cashier in a store, a stranger on the street, a coworker)?"

Anxiety-provoking belief	Examples of questions to ask yourself
"It's important for everyone to like me." (continued)	"Is it possible for everyone to like me?" "Can I think of a person I know whom *everybody* likes?" "Can I think of a person I know whom *nobody* likes?" "Isn't it true that the very things that will make me likable to some people will make me less likable to others (since people tend to like others who are similar to them)?"
"Everything must be neat and tidy. It's important that everything be in its place. If I let even a few things get out of place, everything will turn to chaos."	"Do I have any evidence that letting a few things go will lead to chaos?" "What will happen if a few things are out of order?" "Could I survive feeling uncomfortable for a while because a few items at home are out of place?"

be absolutely terrible and completely unmanageable. Often, when we anticipate some negative event, we assume that it will be awful and that we'd be unable to cope—but we stop short of imagining what it will actually be like and just how we'll react if it were to occur. Decatastrophizing involves taking your catastrophic thoughts to this next stage, thereby taking away their power.

Decatastrophizing involves asking yourself two simple questions:

1. Realistically, what is the worst that could happen?

2. How could I cope with that?

The goal is to discover that the worst is not all that bad and that there's an excellent chance you will be able to cope with most situations that are likely to come up in your life. Here are some examples of how decatastrophizing can be used to fight catastrophic thinking:

Catastrophic thought: "It would be awful to faint during a panic attack."

Decatastrophizing: "What would actually happen if I fainted? Well, I probably would be unconscious for a few seconds and would then regain consciousness. People would probably help me. It might be embarrassing, but that feeling would pass. I guess it wouldn't be the end of the world."

Catastrophic thought: "It would be terrible if I said something stupid in front of others."

Decatastrophizing: "So what if I say something stupid? People say stupid things all the time, and often they don't even seem to care. If I were to say something stupid, a few people might notice, and others might not. Some people might comment on it, and that would be the end of it. It probably wouldn't matter a few minutes later, and it certainly wouldn't matter the next day or the next week."

Catastrophic thought: "It would be awful if my car wasn't fixed by the time the mechanic said it would be ready."

Decatastrophizing: "What would happen if my car wasn't ready? Why would that be such a problem? Could I cope with it? Well, if it's not ready, it would be inconvenient. I would have to get a ride with someone else or take public transportation to work. I could live with that for a few more days if I had to."

Catastrophic thought: "It's terrible to have an intrusive, inappropriate sexual or aggressive thought about another person."

Decatastrophizing: "What is the consequence of having such a thought? Thoughts don't equal actions. Also, the more I try to fight my thoughts, the worse they get. I should just let my thoughts happen. The worst that will occur is that I'll feel uncomfortable. That would be okay. Everyone has inappropriate thoughts sometimes, even though they may not talk about them."

Catastrophic thought: "I think I would want to kill myself if I lost my job."

Decatastrophizing: "How could I cope with losing my job? It would be difficult, but I could live off my credit cards, or with help from relatives, until I found a new job. I could apply for all sorts of positions, or I could even go back to school. I recently read that the typical person changes jobs every 3 or 4 years. If others are able to find a new job that often, then I should be able to find one as well."

Pie Charting

A pie chart can be an effective way of reevaluating your predictions and combating probability overestimations. The benefit of a pie chart is that it always adds up to 100% no matter how many things you add to it. Take a look at Form 6.2 or just draw a circle on a piece of paper. Now take a moment to consider how probable you think your feared outcome is. For most people with anxiety problems, the answer is usually quite high . . . if not 100%. Jot this number down somewhere outside the circle.

Now start estimating how likely *other* outcomes might be and start adding them to your pie chart. You don't need to be incredibly precise about making sure each slice of the pie is exactly the right size, but try to be close. Once you have exhausted your list of other possibilities, see how much of the pie remains and put that amount under "revised estimate of probability" beneath the pie chart.

The first pie chart completed by Jacob, the man introduced earlier who worried he was having a stroke whenever he had a headache, is shown in Sample Completed Form 6.2. If he felt a headache coming on, he would assume that he was 90% likely to be having a stroke. After

Pie Chart

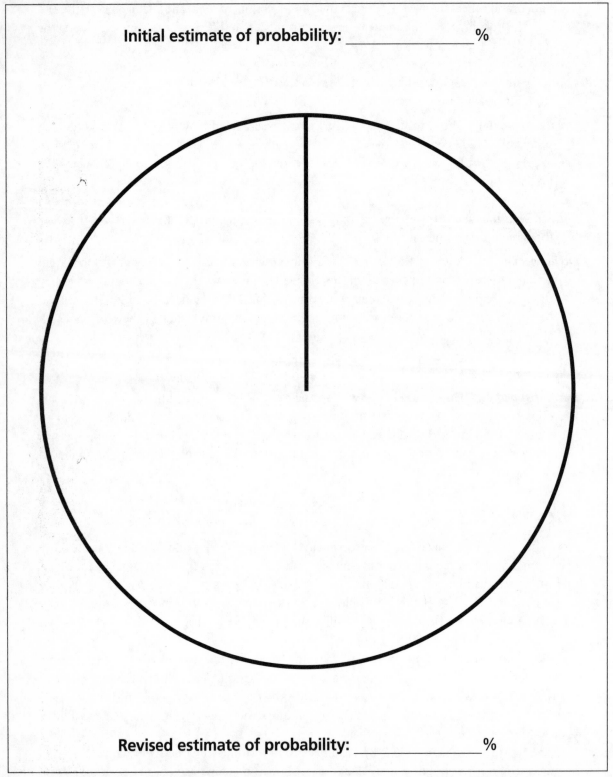

Initial estimate of probability: _____%

Revised estimate of probability: _____%

SAMPLE COMPLETED FORM 6.2 *(Jacob)*

Pie Chart

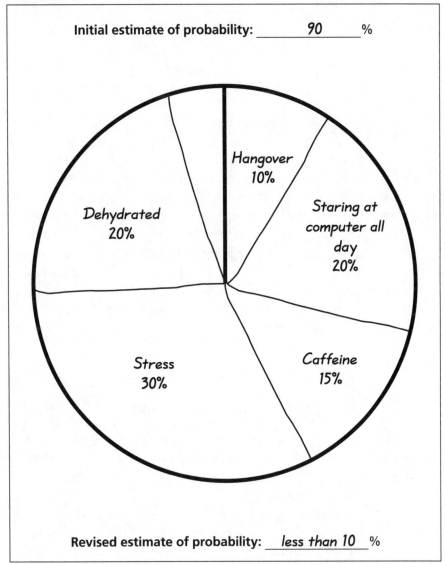

Initial estimate of probability: _____ **90** _____ %

Hangover
10%

Dehydrated
20%

Staring at
computer all
day
20%

Stress
30%

Caffeine
15%

Revised estimate of probability: ___ *less than 10* ___ %

that, Jacob started considering other reasons he might have a headache. The first thought was "a hangover." Jacob didn't drink often, so he estimated that at 10% and filled in a small part of the pie. Next he came up with "staring at the computer all day." As he thought about it, he realized that he does tend to get mild headaches on long days at the office, so he gave that 20% and filled in a larger piece of the pie chart. This continued with "caffeine" (15%), "stress" (30%), and "dehydrated" (20%).

At this point, Jacob stopped filling in the pie chart when he noticed that less than 10% remained and he still had more things he was going to add to the chart that weren't a stroke. He looked carefully at the graph for a few minutes, surprised. In the moments when he has a headache he is so sure that he is having a stroke, but the chart was showing that this was actually very unlikely. He filled out his revised estimate of probability as "less than 10%."

Changing Rigid Rules

Rigid rules are often hard to change because (1) they're difficult to prove or disprove, and (2) they're based on personal values, and we resist changing our values because we don't want to compromise our integrity.

It's up to you to decide which rules and values are worth changing. It's also up to you to decide how much to change a particular rule or value. For example, if you believe that "It's *always* important to make a good impression on others," you wouldn't want to replace that rule with something like "It's *never* important to make a good impression on others." Rather, ask yourself questions that will help you become more flexible with respect to this rule. You might ask whether it's even possible to make a good impression on other people all the time. What are the costs of always having to look good in front of others? Are the costs worth it? Are there some situations in which the consequences of making a bad impression are acceptable? Do other people hold the same values?

By answering questions like these, you may discover that it's quite impossible to meet your own high standards, that other people don't hold the same standards, and that the costs of trying to meet your standards far outweigh the benefits. Just by loosening up your expectations and rules, you may find that you are able to decrease your anxiety.

Changing Core Beliefs

As we mentioned earlier, negative core beliefs represent the most deeply held type of anxiety-related thinking. However, like all beliefs, core beliefs are not facts, and they can be challenged. If you identified one or more negative core beliefs that contribute to your own anxiety (see Form 5.2), try to challenge them. The strategies for changing core beliefs are similar to those for changing other types of negative thinking.

First, identify some alternative core beliefs. If you believe that you're incompetent, for example, you might consider the alternative belief that you're competent. When examining labels such as "competent" and "incompetent," try to define your terms. What does it mean to you to be considered incompetent or competent? This is a first step in gathering evidence to challenge your negative core beliefs.

The next step is to start seeking evidence. Remember, your natural tendency will be to notice information that confirms your negative core belief. Continuing with our example, if you're convinced that you're incompetent, it will be very easy to notice and remember the mistakes you make and much more difficult to notice and remember the competent things you do. Therefore, it can be useful to start keeping a Positive Data Log (see Form 6.3), a diary in which you record each time something happens that disproves your negative core belief. It's a good idea to fill this in throughout the day and to review the information you record on a regular basis. Over time, collecting this information, along with using the other strategies in this chapter, will chip away at your negative core beliefs. (Photocopy the form if needed or download and print extra copies; see the end of the Contents for information.)

FORM 6.3
Positive Data Log

Negative core belief:	
Day and time	**Information that disconfirms my negative core belief**

Troubleshooting

Although the strategies described in this chapter are effective tools for reducing anxiety, obstacles sometimes arise along the way. Here are some of the most common problems that may come up, along with possible solutions.

Problem: "Writing down my thoughts makes me more anxious because it keeps me focused on my anxiety triggers."

Solution: As you'll learn in Chapter 8, repeated exposure to situations that trigger your anxiety should lead to a decrease in anxiety over the long term. Keep completing your Anxiety Thought Records and the process should get easier over time.

Problem: "I hate filling out forms. It reminds me of being in school."

Solution: Even this isn't a problem. The main purpose of the forms is to help you think differently about the situations you fear. If you can do that better without the forms, or by using some other strategy (such as using a diary or audio-recording your responses instead of writing them down), that's fine. Another option is to simplify the forms. Maybe you'd like to develop your own Anxiety Thought Record with just two columns: one for your anxiety-related thoughts and one for your more realistic thoughts.

But before giving up on the forms, try to complete them a few times to see if they become more helpful over time.

Problem: "When I'm feeling anxious, I'm too wound up to complete the forms."

Solution: If you know you're going to have to enter an anxiety-provoking situation, try using the strategies and completing an Anxiety Thought Record *before* entering the situation and before your anxiety has had a chance to peak. Or complete the form later, after your anxiety has decreased. This will provide you with an opportunity to work through what you might have said to yourself when your anxiety was at its peak, which should help you the next time you find yourself in the situation.

Problem: "I used the cognitive strategies to challenge my negative thoughts, but there was no change in my anxiety."

Solution: It often takes a while for the cognitive strategies to start working. At first, they may seem superficial, obvious, or silly. With practice, however, the new nonanxious thoughts should become stronger and the anxiety-provoking thoughts should weaken. If you don't see a shift in your anxiety, consider the possibility that the thoughts you're working on are not the ones that are most closely related to your anxiety. Are there other thoughts that may be more relevant? It's possible too that there is additional evidence you haven't considered. You may need to dig deeper to find additional evidence to challenge your anxiety-related thoughts. Someone else (who doesn't share the same thoughts) may be able to help you come up with additional evidence.

If your anxiety remains high after trying the strategies in this chapter, don't be discouraged! You'll learn many other techniques as you work your way through this book.

Problem: "I'm not experiencing any anxiety lately because I avoid the situations I fear. So I have nothing to record on my Anxiety Thought Record."

Solution: Well, you need some anxiety in order to work through an Anxiety Thought Record. Try confronting situations that arouse at least some anxiety if you're not ready to face your biggest fears yet.

Conclusion

Changing negative thinking begins with viewing one's thoughts as guesses about the way things may be rather than as facts. Other key steps include (1) becoming more aware of our anxiety-related thoughts, (2) considering more balanced, alternative interpretations and predictions, and (3) evaluating the evidence for and against the available interpretations to come up with a realistic way of looking at the situation. Ups and downs may occur when using these strategies, but most people experience a significant drop in anxiety after learning to challenge their anxiety-provoking beliefs. With practice, you will too.

7

changing thinking patterns by taking action

In the previous chapter you learned about challenging your anxiety-provoking thoughts by weighing the evidence and considering alternative possibilities. Many people find that process is enough to help them start breaking down the thinking patterns underlying their anxiety. But for others it isn't quite enough. That's because many of us learn best through firsthand experience.

In this chapter we will discuss several commonly used experiential strategies to gather the evidence you need to evaluate your negative thoughts. Before you try these strategies, however, we recommend that you work through Chapters 5 and 6. The strategies in this chapter build on concepts discussed in these earlier chapters, and they work best if you use them to test out both your anxiety-provoking predictions and possible alternatives.

Think of it like this: If you have a square peg and see only a round hole, you'll keep trying to jam the square peg where it doesn't fit. You may hit it with a hammer to get it in. You may even try to sand down the edges of the square peg so that it fits in the round hole. But if you saw that there was also a square hole, you'd realize that it fits better in there!

Thought-Challenging Strategies

- **Experiments**
- **Surveying others**
- **Expert feedback**

The same principle applies to our thoughts and beliefs. If we allow ourselves to consider only one possibility, then we typically either try to make any new information fit into that belief or we ignore information that simply doesn't fit. But if we open ourselves to considering the possibility that an alternative might be true—even if we don't yet believe it—then we allow ourselves the ability to see which possibility the evidence supports best.

Experiments

In the previous chapters, we mentioned that changing your anxiety-provoking thoughts involves thinking like a scientist. So, how do scientists make discoveries? They conduct experiments.

A researcher who believes that treating high blood pressure by changing diet and increasing exercise is likely to be more effective than a standard medication treatment might test out this hypothesis by conducting an experiment. She might take a large group of people with high blood pressure and give half of them medication and the other half instructions to change their diet and exercise regimes. If the treatment involving changes to diet and exercise works best, that's a sign that the researcher's hypothesis may be correct. It would also be important to see if the results could be repeated over several studies by several different researchers, since the results of any one study may be due to chance or the specific ways in which the study was designed.

Experiments can also be used to test out your own anxiety-provoking predictions. For example, Leanne's panic attacks tended to be triggered by any activity that made her heart race, like exercise or sex. She was convinced that if she didn't stop exercising or having sex when she started to feel panicky, she would collapse from a heart attack. So she always rested when she noticed her panicky feelings coming on. She eventually stopped exercising and having sex altogether. Leanne believed that sitting down or resting when she felt panicky was the only way to prevent a heart attack and perhaps save her life. When her therapist asked her to come up with an alternative, balanced belief, she acknowledged that another interpretation would be that her panic attacks and racing heart are not dangerous and that sitting down during panic attacks has nothing to do with whether she lives or dies.

Can you think of an experiment that could be designed to test out which of these two beliefs is correct? Well, one option is for Leanne to exercise and then not sit down when she starts to feel panicky. As long as she is physically healthy, which her family doctor has confirmed, there would be little to no risk in trying an experiment like this, and it could show Leanne that she doesn't need to rest when she feels panicky during exercise.

Similar experiments can be designed to test out a whole range of anxiety-related beliefs. The box below and on the next page provides examples of specific predictions that would be likely to lead to anxiety, along with experiments that could be used to test out each prediction.

Now you're ready to plan some of your own experiments. Use the Experiment Record (Form 7.1) to plan an experiment and record your results. In the first column, record an

---

Using Experiments to Challenge Anxious Beliefs

Anxiety-provoking thought	Examples of possible experiments
"I'll get sick if I don't wash my hands after being out in public."	Don't wash your hands for one day and see if you get sick.
"It would be terrible if I were to look anxious in public."	Let yourself purposely look anxious. Put an anxious look on your face, let your hands shake, and put some water on your forehead to simulate sweating. Then go out in public. Do people seem to notice? Do they seem to care? Are there any negative consequences at all, other than your feeling uncomfortable?

Anxiety-provoking thought	Examples of possible experiments
"I phone my partner every hour during the day because I always need to know where she is in case something terrible happens to one of us."	Try *not* calling your partner for one day. Other than feeling uncomfortable, does anything bad happen?
"If I ask others for directions, they will think I'm stupid."	Stand in a public place for an hour and ask everyone who walks by for directions. Is there any indication that most of them think you're stupid?
"If I go out on a date with a man, he will attack me."	Try going out on a date (of course, take the precautions that most people would take: make sure you know something about the person and have the first date in a public place). Do you get attacked?
"If I make a left turn in the car, I will get hit by another driver."	Try making lots of left turns for an hour or so and see what happens.

anxiety-provoking thought or prediction. In the second column, list one or more alternative (non-anxiety-provoking) thoughts or predictions. In the third column, describe the experiment you will conduct to test out whether the belief recorded in column 1 is accurate. In the fourth column, record the outcome of your experiment, and rate your anxiety from 0 (none) to 100 (extreme) now that you have thought about the results of the experiment. What actually occurred? What evidence did you gain? Did your prediction come true? What did you learn from the experiment? What did it tell you about the accuracy of your original prediction? Now record a more accurate thought, based on the results of your experiment, in the box at the bottom of the Experiment Record.

Did my expectations actually come true?

Make it a point to conduct several experiments each week and complete an Experiment Record each time (photocopy or download and print extra forms; see the end of the Contents for information).

Surveying Others

Surveying a group of people can be an easy way to gather unbiased information about a range of different anxiety-related thoughts and can be especially useful if your thoughts tend to be guesses about what others are thinking or assuming. Bindi, the socially anxious university student we've been following, agreed that she regularly engaged in "mind-reading"—assuming that she knew what people thought of her. Whenever she gave a presentation in class, she assumed

Experiment Record

Anxiety-provoking thoughts and predictions	Alternative thoughts and predictions	Experiment description	Evidence and realistic conclusions/Anxiety after completing experiment (0–100)

Record a more accurate thought based on the results of your experiment:

that "They all think that I don't know what I'm talking about." After one short presentation, she asked a few of the students in her class how they thought it went. To her surprise, they all gave very positive feedback. One classmate even told her, "I didn't really understand that topic until you explained it so much better than the professor ever did."

Surveys can also be helpful in gathering realistic information about how common certain types of beliefs are. Jacqui, the woman you've met who had intrusive thoughts about harming her newborn child, also thought a survey would be helpful. Her therapist, Ruby, had told her that these sorts of thoughts are actually quite common among new mothers, even those without obsessive–compulsive difficulties. Jacqui liked and trusted Ruby as a therapist but just couldn't believe that it was true. So Jacqui decided to anonymously post "I know this is weird, but have any of you had thoughts or images pop into your mind about harming your child?" to a "New Moms" forum online. Jacqui was astonished that within a few hours hundreds of moms had replied. A few people made some mean-spirited comments—not unusual for the Internet these days—but most of them said that they had. A few people were thankful that Jacqui brought up the question . . . they also thought they were the only ones! These survey results really affected Jacqui. In particular, she had two realizations that she found incredibly helpful:

"Can I really be a bad mom if I'm having the same thoughts as all of these other moms?"

"So many moms have these kinds of thoughts and they've never harmed their babies. What makes me any different?"

Using Form 7.2, try to develop a survey that you could use to test some of your assumptions. The form may not be perfect for every type of survey, so feel free to modify it as necessary. Then record your anxiety-related prediction of what the survey will say and go talk to people to see if your negative prediction matches the results of the survey.

Collecting Expert Feedback

Getting expert feedback is quite similar to taking surveys in many ways, but instead of asking a bunch of "regular" people, the focus is on identifying a small number of people who are clearly experts to provide you with information or feedback. Be sure to select experts who are as unbiased as possible and have the credentials to back up their responses. A scientist at the U.S. National Weather Service, for example, would be a valuable and unbiased expert source of information on how dangerous a thunderstorm system will be. Asking someone without any particular credentials who runs a health blog might not be a good choice, because you can't be sure of how much the person knows.

As an example, one former client was terrified of swimming in the ocean for fear of encountering sharks. She understood that it might just seem like there are a lot of shark attacks because she repeatedly Googled "shark attack," so she developed a list of experts she could e-mail to ask how common shark attacks are. The experts she e-mailed included a scientist at the local aquarium, which had sharks, a university-based marine biologist who studied sharks, and the lifeguard organization from an Australian TV show called *Bondi Beach*. She didn't hear back

Survey Form

What questions will you ask the people you are surveying?

1. _____

2. _____

3. _____

What does your anxious mind think the results will be?

Record the survey responses below:

What were the results of your survey?

from the lifeguards, but both the scientist from the aquarium and the university marine biologist did respond. They both said that shark attacks are extremely rare, and the aquarium scientist also gave her some other statistics to put the risk into context. Did you know that in the United States almost 11,000 people are injured by buckets or pails each year, as compared with 13 people injured by sharks?

Troubleshooting

Although the strategies described in this chapter are usually effective for reducing anxiety, obstacles sometimes arise along the way. Here is one of the most common problems that may come up, along with some possible solutions.

Problem: "I would be too embarrassed to do a survey or ask for expert feedback."

Solution: If fear of embarrassment is too strong for you right now, consider doing an anonymous survey online or creating a new e-mail address to contact the expert. Perhaps a loved one could help out by asking people the survey questions on your behalf. Or best of all, you could design an experiment to test what happens if you did ask someone a survey question or contacted an expert!

Conclusion

Many people find the "proof" they obtain through real-life experience to be much more convincing than rationally challenging their own thoughts. Evidence that you can see with your own eyes can be very hard to dismiss, especially if you've allowed yourself to consider the chance that an alternative might be possible—that you might have a square hole too.

Some of the action-oriented techniques for testing your thoughts include creating experiments, surveying people, seeking expert feedback, and pie charting. All of these are fairly simple techniques, especially if you plan them in advance. What kind of experiment would let you definitively test whether your anxiety-related beliefs are correct? How could I get unbiased information to see whether my assumptions are valid? Not every technique will fit your specific thoughts and beliefs, and sometimes the results will be unclear. If they are, be like a detective or a scientist and try to improve your experiment or survey to get a clearer answer!

8

introduction to confronting your fears

In 1999, Dr. David Satcher, then U.S. surgeon general, produced perhaps the most complete review of mental health and treatment ever published. In it, he stated that the most important and critical part of treatment for anxiety is "exposure to the stimuli or situations that provoke anxiety"—in other words, facing your fears. Experts in the treatment of anxiety call this *exposure*. In the two decades since Dr. Satcher's report, the importance of doing exposure has not changed.

> **Exposure is the most powerful strategy for overcoming fears!**

In this chapter, you'll learn about the elements of planning and conducting your own exposures. Read this chapter to understand what exposure is and how exposures should be conducted in general. The subsequent chapters will address using exposures for different kinds of anxiety problems. Chapter 9 provides important additional tips for exposures to *objects and situations* that cause you anxiety; Chapter 10 describes exposure to fearful *thoughts*; and Chapter 11 discusses exposure to fearful *sensations* in your body. The key to all of these different types of exposure is to *experience your emotions* (for example, fear and anxiety)—not just simply to experience the objects, situations, thoughts, or sensations. In each chapter, we'll show you how to develop a step-by-step plan to begin confronting your fears, starting with the easier fears.

Exposure involves confronting your emotions by facing the situations, objects, sensations, or thoughts that trigger your anxiety. Don't try to confront your worst fears immediately or to face all your fears at once! Experts in the treatment of anxiety call that *flooding*. Although it can be effective, it should be done only with the help of an experienced mental health professional. Instead, we recommend *graduated exposure,* starting with your easier fears and then, when you have gained confidence and success in overcoming those fears, gradually moving on to more difficult fears.

Exposure will probably be the most important strategy for your recovery. Unfortunately, it can also be the most difficult strategy because it requires you to do exactly what your mind has been telling you *not* to do. And it only works if you give 100%. So you have to be ready to make a commitment.

Because this can be challenging, we recommend doing another motivational enhancement like the one you did in Chapter 3. Do another cost–benefit analysis using Form 8.1 to help remind yourself of the pros of tackling your anxiety and moving yourself toward an anti-anxiety lifestyle. Then, when you're ready, sign the Exposure Contract on the facing page and rely on it to inspire you when your motivation starts to slip. Print out a copy and carry it with you or post it on the refrigerator if that helps. (Rereading Chapter 3 may also be helpful when your motivation needs a boost.)

FORM 8.1

Costs and Benefits of Using This Program

What are your long-term goals and desires? What would you like to do with your life in the next 1 to 3 years?
_____
_____
_____
_____

Now, thinking about your own anxiety and your own life, record the costs and benefits of (1) working through this program and (2) not working through this program.	
Working through the program **(0–100 importance)**	**Not working through the program** **(–100–0 importance)**
Pros _____ (___) _____ (___) _____ (___) _____ (___)	*Pros* _____ (___) _____ (___) _____ (___) _____ (___)
Cons _____ (___) _____ (___) _____ (___) _____ (___)	*Cons* _____ (___) _____ (___) _____ (___) _____ (___)

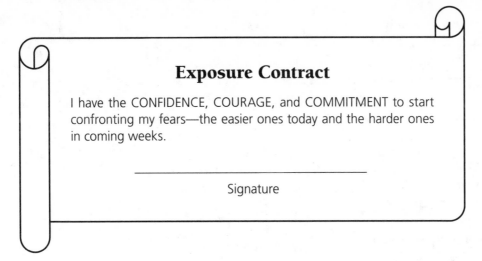

Exposure Contract

I have the CONFIDENCE, COURAGE, and COMMITMENT to start confronting my fears—the easier ones today and the harder ones in coming weeks.

_____

Signature

How Does Exposure Work?

Reading Joseph's story will help you understand how exposure works and how successful it can be. In telling his story, we've interjected some questions for you to think about.

Joseph and the Diving Board

Joseph celebrated his 16th birthday with his family and friends at a public pool in a nearby big city. This pool had been built for international competition, so it had a full range of diving platforms. But Joseph, who grew up in a small town a couple hours away, had never been on a diving board more than a couple feet off the ground. He couldn't wait, because he had heard stories from his older brother about having fun jumping from the diving boards dozens of times.

Joseph eagerly climbed the ladder to the 10-foot-high platform—but then he looked down. He felt like he was a mile in the air, and the water no longer seemed as if it would be soft to land in. He desperately wanted to turn around and head back down the ladder.

How might turning around and escaping his fear make Joseph feel about himself?

Fortunately, Joseph's family and friends were in the water, encouraging him to jump. Even though he was scared, he mustered up his courage and jumped, screaming in terror the whole way down. After the splash, he felt astonished that he was still alive. His first thought was that he never wanted to do that again. But he watched the other kids having fun jumping from the diving board, and his family encouraged him to try it again. As he climbed back up, he still felt afraid, but not as much as last time, which seemed strange. He found it a little easier to jump the second time. And it wasn't as scary on the way down. The third time was even better, and so was the fourth. By the fifth time, he was racing up the ladder and letting out a shout of *"Woo-hoo!"* as he flung himself into the water.

Joseph didn't know it, but he was doing exposure therapy. By repeatedly confronting his fear, he lost the feeling of terror when standing on the diving board. Later that day he climbed up to the 5-meter (about 15-foot) board. Was he scared? You bet! But not quite as scared as the first time he had stood on the lowest platform. After a few jumps, he lost his fear and just enjoyed himself. The same process happened a few weeks later when he tried the 7.5-meter platform.

> *If Joseph turned around and escaped his fear, would he be more or less likely to try diving again?*

> *Have you had an experience like this where you were initially scared but felt better after trying something a few times?*

> **By confronting his fears again and again, Joseph made them gradually disappear, and he actually began to enjoy himself.**

This is graduated exposure: confronting your fears gradually, starting with easier situations and building up to harder ones as your anxiety starts to diminish.

Why Does Exposure Work?

Psychologists have studied exposure therapy since the 1960s. They have found that the more we confront something, the less we tend to react to it. Can you remember a really scary movie you saw, perhaps a few years back? Do you think it would have been as scary if you had watched it again the next day? How about a third time? A fourth time? A tenth? It's human nature to get used to things over time. By practicing exposure to the situations you fear, you will get used to them, just as Joseph did.

Why does exposure work? Psychological researchers used to believe that when you repeatedly exposed yourself to the things that provoked your fears, your previous learning that a situation was dangerous would slowly fade away. They called this "extinction," and it originally came from the studies of Pavlov's dogs. In these classic experiments, Dr. Pavlov would ring a bell every time he fed his dogs, and before long the dogs salivated whenever they heard the bell, even if there was no food. The dogs learned that "bell = food." This is how a lot of fears are learned as well. If we have a negative experience in a situation, we can learn to see the situation as dangerous. Being frightened when his father had a headache and then collapsed due to a stroke led Jacob to "learn" that headaches are dangerous.

More importantly for us, Dr. Pavlov also noticed in his experiments that if he rang the bell enough times without giving his dogs any food, the "bell = food" learning would disappear and the dogs would no longer salivate at the sound of the bell. This led us to believe that learned fears would also fade away when people did exposures. But modern experiments show us that it is a little more complicated. Rather than extinguishing old learning, exposure therapy creates *new* safety learning. When the new safety learning becomes strong enough, it inhibits, but doesn't get rid of, the old danger learning.

One important thing about this distinction is that danger learning tends to be more durable than safety learning. This makes sense; our brains tend to err on the side of caution in order to try to keep us safe. If we encounter the things we previously feared again unexpectedly or in new situations, the danger learning is more likely to take over rather than the safety learning. And this is why psychologists and other mental health professionals know that it is essential to practice exposures over and over in all sorts of new situations, so that it is more likely that the new safety learning will inhibit the old danger learning. Incidentally, this is also why people who have had many positive experiences with something (such as many happy times playing with a dog) are less likely to develop fears involving that thing after one bad experience (like later being bitten by a dog).

Exposure allows us to learn that our feared outcome won't necessarily come to pass. In the last chapters, you learned strategies for changing your anxiety-related thoughts. But it's one thing to *tell* yourself that something bad isn't going to happen (or that it won't be as bad as you think if it does happen) and another thing entirely to *learn that it's true through direct experience.* Remember Joseph when he first stood on the edge of the diving board? What do you think he was expecting to happen if he jumped? He probably thought he would feel horrible and that he might get hurt or die. What do you think he thought after he jumped the first time? Probably that it felt horrible, but that he didn't get hurt or die. What about the next time? Not so horrible, didn't get hurt or die, and a little exhilarating. Next time: "This is fun! Why was I so scared before?" He proved his anxious thoughts wrong.

Exposure has the added benefit of promoting confidence and courage. Each time you successfully confront your fears, you give yourself an extra boost of self-confidence. You tell yourself, "I did it, and I can do it again." And you start to feel that you can try other things you've been avoiding. You're getting control of your anxiety—and your life! This feeling of confidence is almost addictive. The more you overcome, the more you want to push yourself further. It's just like an athlete who turns in her personal best performance. She knows she can do it, she believes that she can do even better, and she wants to try even harder next time. And so will you.

Creating an Exposure Plan

The first step in beginning exposure is to create a list of the triggers that cause you to feel anxious. You can use the situations you listed on the forms in Chapter 2 as a start. Then, using Form 8.2, list up to 10 situations, objects, physical sensations, or thoughts/memories that cause you fear or discomfort or that you avoid because of your anxiety. Make sure to list some that cause less fear and some that cause more. You can break apart some triggers into easier and harder parts, such as *seeing a plastic snake* versus *seeing a real snake,* or *going to an empty supermarket* versus *going to the supermarket when it is busy.* If you're working on more than one type of fear, use different forms if that makes it easier for you. In most cases a list of 10 triggers that includes some of your most difficult fears is enough. But feel free to list more. Be as specific as you can in listing the triggers. (Photocopy the form as needed or download and print extra copies; see the end of the Contents for information on downloading.)

Exposure Plan

Rank order	Fear trigger: Situation, object, thought, or sensations	Fear rating (0–100)

Once you've come up with about 10 triggers or objects, go back and rank them in order from 1 (the worst or most frightening trigger) to 10 (the least frightening trigger on the list). Finally, for each trigger, make a rating of how much fear or discomfort you would experience if you were to face it. Rate each situation or object from 0 (wouldn't scare you at all) to 100 (the scariest thing you can imagine).

When you're done, you may find it helpful to write out the list again, in order of difficulty, from 1 (the hardest situation or object) to 10 (the easiest situation or object). Usually it's best if the #1 trigger is something that has a fear rating of 80 to 100 and the #10 trigger has a fear rating of about 30 or 40. This will give you a ladder you can move up as you start to confront more and more difficult triggers, just as Joseph moved up to higher and higher diving platforms. Now, on Form 8.3, rewrite your list in order of difficulty. (Again, photocopy or download and print extra copies as needed.)

Sample Completed Form 8.3 (Jacob) shows an example of an Exposure Plan for Jacob, the man who worries about having a stroke after having seen his father collapse. Jacob becomes very anxious when he has unusual physical sensations that he believes are signs that he is having a stroke or an aneurysm. He's also extremely anxious doing things that he thinks will bring on these physical sensations, especially exercising. Finally, he also notices that he gets anxious when things remind him of his health emergencies, like remembering his father's stroke or being in hospitals.

Remember Jacqui, the new mother who has been having intrusive thoughts about accidentally harming her new daughter? Her Exposure Plan focuses on two types of things: the thoughts themselves and situations or objects that seem to cause those thoughts to pop into her mind. Take a look at Jacqui's Exposure Plan on Sample Completed Form 8.3 (Jacqui).

Carrying Out Your Exposure Plan

In the next three chapters we'll give you more specific details about how you can conduct exposures to situations or objects, thoughts or memories, and physical sensations. Please read those chapters that were identified in your treatment plan (Chapter 4) as being important for you before beginning your exposures. All exposure exercises have aspects in common that we will discuss here.

Choosing a Good Exposure Practice

Remember, the goal is generally to start with easier exposures and then work your way up to the more difficult ones when you feel ready. It may seem daunting at first, but you can do this—many others before you have successfully done it. Look over your plan. Are triggers 10 or 9 things that you could easily face? Are they exposures that would cause *some* anxiety, but not be overwhelming? Are there items higher on your list that you feel ready to try? If so, that's fine too (it's not necessary to start at the bottom of your list or even to go in order).

Carefully select your first exposure, then take the steps on page 137 to ensure that you get as much benefit as possible from it.

Exposure Plan in Order of Difficulty

Rank order	Fear trigger: Situation, object, thought, or sensations	Fear rating (0–100)
1		
2		
3		
4		
5		
6		
7		
8		
9		
10		

Exposure Plan in Order of Difficulty

Rank order	Fear trigger: Situation, object, thought, or sensations	Fear rating (0–100)
1	Feeling a sudden headache	100
2	Feeling my heart race	95
3	Being at the hospital	90
4	Thinking about when Dad had his stroke	80
5	Seeing people who look like they have had a stroke	70
6	Doing a vigorous workout	60
7	Feeling lightheaded	55
8	Running	50
9	Blurry vision or "eye tracers" or anything funny with my vision	40
10	Doing a light workout	30

Exposure Plan in Order of Difficulty

Rank order	Fear trigger: Situation, object, thought, or sensations	Fear rating (0–100)
1	Having anything around that could potentially be a weapon (like a pencil) when I'm alone with my daughter	90
2	Changing my daughter's diaper when alone	85
3	Having thoughts that I might have poisoned my daughter	85
4	Having thoughts that I might have touched my daughter	80
5	Changing my daughter's diaper when my partner is around	80
6	Driving on the freeway with daughter	60
7	Hearing my daughter cry at night—worry I did something wrong	50
8	Dropping my daughter off at my in-laws'—worry they will find something that looks like an injury	50
9	Driving in my car on regular streets with daughter	40
10	Taking daughter to physician—worry she will find something that looks like an injury	40

1. **Determine whether the trigger you plan to start with is (a) an object or situation, (b) a thought, or (c) a physical sensation.** It's important to know what kind of trigger you're addressing because your exposure should be as similar as possible to the trigger. If your anxiety goes up when going to specific places such as the grocery store, for example, you should plan to do an exposure at that place. Doing an exposure where you imagine that you are going to that place is probably not going to be very helpful. If your anxiety is related to a certain memory, such as when you were in an earthquake, you should work on doing exposures to that memory. Look over your Exposure Plan and decide whether each of the triggers is an object or situation (Chapter 9), a mental experience (Chapter 10), or a physical sensation (Chapter 11), and plan to do an exposure that most closely matches each trigger.

2. **Identify exactly how you're going to arrange the exposure.** This is important. If you can't *arrange* to do the exposure, you can't *do* the exposure! Take some time to figure out exactly how you can make it happen. Don't leave it to chance or "wing it" to see what happens. If your exposure involves touching things in the bathroom that you fear might be covered in germs, make sure you have a private bathroom that you can use. If it involves being around snakes, check to see if your local zoo has a snake exhibit. If it involves going somewhere that reminds you of a previous assault, choose a safe but similar place where you can spend some time. A bit of planning will help you to get the most out of your exposure.

For exposures that involve finding a safe but similar place, you will need to distinguish between what *is* safe and what *feels* safe. For someone with a height phobia, for example, sitting on a sturdy balcony or standing near a window in a high-rise building is safe even if it doesn't feel safe. Sitting on the rail around a balcony, on the other hand, isn't safe (and probably doesn't feel safe either). Many people can be honest with themselves about whether something is unsafe or just feels unsafe. If you're having trouble with this distinction, ask a family member, friend, coworker, or therapist to help you decide.

3. **Before you begin, identify your anxiety-provoking thoughts so you can test them out.** Identify your anxiety-provoking thoughts before you begin, using the strategies you learned in Chapter 7. For someone doing an exposure to traumatic memories of a horrible earthquake, an anxiety-provoking thought might be "If I think about it, I'll lose control of my emotions." For someone doing an exposure involving locking the door only once and not checking it, an anxiety-provoking thought might be "Someone might break in and kill my family, and it would be my fault." Someone doing an exposure to feeling his heart racing might have the thought "I might have a heart attack and die."

When you have identified your anxiety-provoking thought, try to also identify an "alternative thought." After you have completed the practice, reflect on the exposure and identify whether the anxiety-provoking thought or the alternative thought is true (we will come back to this).

4. **Set specific goals.** Those of us with anxiety problems are often our own harshest critics. We sometimes don't give ourselves credit for our successes, focusing instead on what went wrong or what we didn't do. So it's useful to set some goals for the exposure. Then you can look back afterward and see whether you met them.

How can you figure out how to set your goals?

- They should be realistic but challenging.

- They should focus on specific actions, not feelings.

- They should be measurable (in many cases, this means that someone else should be able to watch and tell you whether you met your goal).

- The achievement of the goal should be completely under your control.

Some examples of helpful goals, as well as some not-so-helpful goals, are listed in the following box.

Helpful versus Unhelpful Goals

Goal	Good or bad	Why
To ask someone out on a date	✓	This goal is very clear, challenging but realistic, and completely under your control. You either ask or you don't.
To get a date	✗	While this goal is clear and challenging, it isn't under your control. The person could say no. He or she could be married, not ready to date, or simply not interested.
Not to feel anxious while making a presentation at work	✗	This goal focuses on feelings, not actions. It isn't realistic right now to expect that you won't feel anxious. The more often you practice, the less anxious you will feel. Limit your goals to things you do, not things you feel.
To make it through my entire presentation	✓	This goal is under your control. It is up to you whether to stop. It is an action, and it is something that someone else could measure.

Now that you better understand what kind of goal to set, take a moment to think about your upcoming exposure. What do you feel would be a good, specific, realistic though challenging, action-oriented goal that is completely within your control? Remember to focus on actions rather than feelings. Write your goal below.

My Goal for the Exposure Exercise

_____

---

5. **Begin the exposure.** You've arranged the exposure, identified your anxious thoughts and considered some alternatives, and set your goals. Now it's time to actually do the exposure. Expect some anxiety the first few times (after all, if you weren't anxious you wouldn't be doing this!). Remember to keep the big picture in mind—the small investment you're making now will pay great dividends in the near future.

While you're doing the exposure, pay attention every few moments to how scared or uncomfortable you're feeling. If it's useful, keep track of it on a 0–100 scale, with higher scores meaning more fear. Don't get discouraged. Though you may notice your anxiety increasing initially, or maybe staying the same, if you stick with the exposure for long enough, your level of fear will start to come down. On page 140 you can see the graph of Callum's fear ratings during a 5-minute exposure to riding on a "sea taxi"—a small ferry that takes people across a river or harbor—to confront his fears of being trapped and unable to escape. Callum was very anxious at first, but as you can see, as the trip progressed his anxiety level dropped quickly.

Your fear ratings will also drop after the beginning of an exposure and will usually come down more each time you repeat the same exposure. Remember how that happened for Joseph when he kept jumping off the diving board? Look at the bottom graph on page 140 and you'll see how each time Callum rode the sea taxi his anxiety didn't get as high as the previous time, and it came down more quickly.

Finishing Your Exposure and Reviewing Your Goal

Once you have completed the exposure, congratulate yourself! You've begun the hardest, but most powerful, technique for overcoming your anxiety. Facing your fears takes a lot of courage and resilience. You should be proud of yourself.

When you get to the point where you're pleased with your accomplishments, you may want to look back at the exposure. Did you meet the goal you wrote down? Resist the temptation to *qualify* whether or not you met the goal—as in *"Yes, but . . . "* The anxious mind wants to forget or ignore successes and focus on failures. The image on page 141 shows some examples of qualifications/equivocations followed by statements you can use to challenge such thoughts.

Finally, now is a good time to review the anxiety-provoking thoughts you had before and during the exposure. Compare them to what actually happened. This is important! It will give you extra courage the next time you do this exposure. Use it to remind yourself that while you *expected* something terrible to happen, what *really* happened wasn't nearly as bad as you expected. In fact, most people are surprised by how well things turned out. Rather than feeling awful and miserable the whole time, it sometimes turns out to be quite enjoyable.

That was exactly Robin's experience when she started doing exposures. Robin had a fear of vomiting, and for years she had not gone out for a meal, either at restaurants or at friends' houses. She was terrified that the food would not be cooked properly or would be prepared in an unsanitary way and that she would develop food poisoning and throw up.

Part of Robin's exposure plan was to eat dinner at a nice restaurant with some of her friends. Admittedly, she first checked with the health department to see if the restaurant had received any complaints or poor inspection reports. The report was clean, but she still felt nervous about going. Robin expected to have a terrible time since she was sure she'd be nervous and on guard

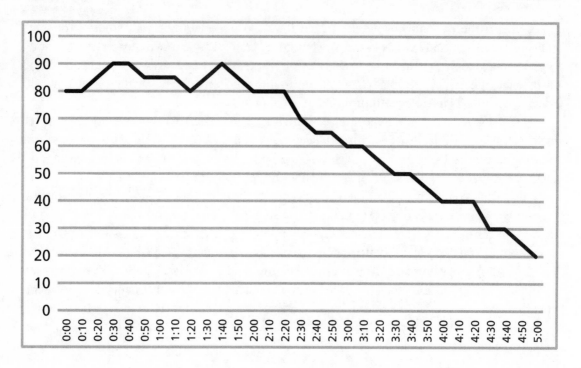

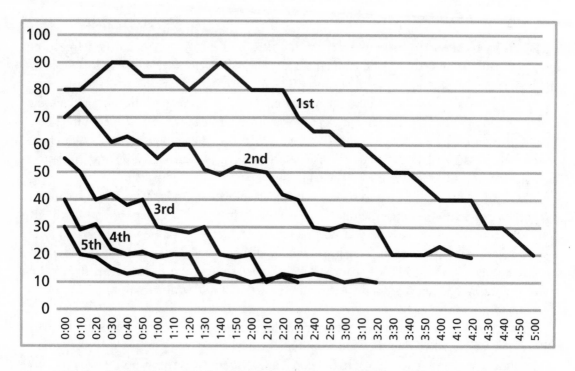

Graph of Callum's fear ratings during a 5-minute exposure riding on a sea taxi, going down over one (top) and multiple (bottom) exposures.

during the whole meal. She also expected to get sick, if not from the food, then from worrying so much. With a little encouragement from her best friend, Robin went to the restaurant.

While she felt moderately scared when reading the menu and ordering her meal, Robin soon realized that she was having such a fun time with her friends that she had completely stopped worrying about the possibility of getting sick. Realizing that she didn't get sick and that in fact she had a lot of fun, Robin started trying more and more different exposures, which helped to boost her enthusiasm and courage.

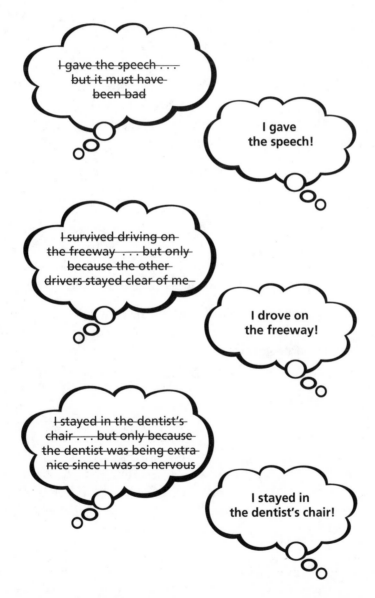

Examples of qualifications/equivocations versus fair review of goals met.

Continuing with Exposure Therapy

If you're wondering what you should do after completing your first exposure, the best thing is to do the same (or a similar) exposure a few more times. Doing an exposure just once usually won't make an impact on your anxiety over the long term. Joseph, the 16-year-old on the diving board, would have remained scared if he had jumped off only once. What got him over his fear was jumping off the diving board many times. Keep practicing over and over until your first exposure doesn't cause you as much anxiety as it did before. We usually recommend practicing each exposure until it no longer causes your anxiety to go above 30 or 40. When you feel ready to move on to a more difficult exposure, do it and continue until it comes down to a 30 or 40.

In addition, plan to practice each exposure as often (frequency), as long (duration), and in as many similar situations (variety) as possible. Here are the key guidelines to keep in mind as you plan exposure practices:

■ **Frequency:** Exposure works best when practices are carried out *frequently*. In other words, it's better to practice four or five times per day rather than once per week. If exposures are too spread out, each time will be like starting over. The more frequently you do exposures, and the closer together they are to each other, the more effective they will be.

■ **Duration:** Exposure is most effective when practices are *prolonged*. Ideally, your practices should last long enough for your fear to decrease to a mild level, or until you learn that your anxiety-provoking predictions don't come true. However, even if your fear doesn't come down within a given practice, don't give up—you should still see improvement across practices. Don't try to rush through your exposure "just to get it over with" . . . try to keep going for a few more minutes, just to make sure your anxiety doesn't spring back up. For most situations, you should practice your exposures again and again for between 30 minutes and a few hours.

■ **Variety:** Practice your exposures in as many different situations and at as many different times as possible. If you are doing driving exposures, try many different streets in several neighborhoods. Practice in the morning, in the afternoon, and at night. Practice in clear weather, and when it's raining. If possible, practice in different cars. The idea is to prepare for any situation that might come up so that you will always have "safety learning" to counteract the old "danger learning."

■ **Other key points:** Early on, you should engage in exposures that are *predictable* (in other words, you know what to expect), as well as under your *control* (as opposed to being forced to confront a feared situation against your will). Over time, you can introduce exposures to unpredictable and uncertain situations, and situations where you have less control over what happens. In fact, as you will see in Chapter 10, *exposure to uncertainty* can be used to get over a fear of uncertain situations.

In an ideal world, you would practice your exposures every day doing as many back-to-back exposures as you could in a variety of situations. Bindi, the socially anxious university student from a small rural town (described in the Introduction), decided that one of her first exposures would be to have "small-talk" conversations with strangers. Knowing the importance of duration, frequency, and variety, she decided that she would try to initiate small-talk conversations with different strangers every day for a full week. To make sure she got the **duration** part, she decided that each small-talk conversation would go on for at least 10 minutes, unless of course the person she was talking to had to leave! For **frequency,** she decided that each day she would initiate four conversations within a 1-hour period. Finally, for **variety,** Bindi decided to mix up the "when," the "where," and the "who." Some days she would do her exposures in the morning before class, other days in the afternoon, and sometimes in the evening. She decided to sometimes initiate conversations with women, sometimes with men, and sometimes with both; in class, on campus, or out in the community; with professors, with staff, or with fellow students.

Obviously some exposures might be more difficult to arrange very often—like those for fear of flying—because of time and expense. That's all right! Just use the **duration, frequency, and variety** principles as best you can. If you are taking a flight for your exposure, see if you can book an itinerary that has as many layovers as possible so you can experience many takeoffs and landings (**frequency**) on 1-hour flights (**duration**) on different airplanes or in different parts of the airplane (**variety**).

When your fear has decreased to a level where you are willing to try something more difficult, that's your signal to move on. There are two ways of proceeding:

1. Just as Joseph moved up to the 5-meter diving board, you could start moving up to the more difficult situations on your Exposure Plan.

2. Start eliminating any actions you take, or things you keep with you, that make you feel safer during the exposures. We call these *safety behaviors*. They'll be discussed in the next section.

Removing Safety Behaviors

Safety behaviors are *behaviors,* or sometimes *objects* or *thoughts,* that we use to control our anxiety when we face situations we fear. Technically, it would be more accurate to call them "false safety behaviors." They're false because they don't actually protect us from any danger; they just make us *feel* safer.

Safety Behaviors and Objects

An example of a safety behavior would be the compulsive behaviors that people with obsessive–compulsive disorder (OCD) feel compelled to repeat. These include repeatedly washing their hands for fear that they might have become contaminated, checking and rechecking the doors or appliances for fear that they might not have been locked or turned off properly, or repeating any behavior over and over to get rid of an ominous feeling that something bad might happen.

Though these types of behaviors are among the most dramatic, most people with an anxiety problem engage in behaviors that they believe keep them safer. It's not uncommon for people with panic disorder to make sure they keep a water bottle, a cell phone, or a bottle of pills (even an empty pill bottle!) with them at all times. People with agoraphobia often prepare for going out into crowded places by studying maps of buildings or malls so they know where all the exits are. They may take a trusted person out with them to help in case they begin to panic. The list of ways in which people try to manage their anxieties and fears is nearly endless.

The problem with safety behaviors is that they wind up actually strengthening the anxiety and getting in the way of your efforts to reduce it. Take a look at the different experiences of Sully and Sally, who both have panic disorder and agoraphobia.

Sully	Sally
Sully has had panic disorder for about 4 years. During this time he also started avoiding public places where he felt he couldn't get help if he started to panic. This includes any number of places, but he lists malls, arenas, and large crowds as his worst situations.	Sally has had panic disorder for about 5 years. Roughly 3 years ago, she found herself avoiding places with large crowds where she felt she couldn't escape if she started to panic. She isn't quite housebound, but she has an extremely hard time going to any stores, malls, or theaters.
Sully began his exposure plan by going to the mall first thing in the morning on a weekday. He figured that the mall would be nearly empty at this time. Sully knew about the need to eliminate safety behaviors but decided that he absolutely needed to keep his anti-anxiety pills with him in case of an emergency. He did leave his water bottle, which he normally took everywhere, at home. "I will do the exposure, but I need my pills as a safety net . . . just in case," he thought.	Sally began her exposure plan by going to some smaller malls at times when she knew there would be fewer people there. Sally knew about eliminating safety behaviors, so she chose to leave her cell phone at home during the exposure. She also made sure to remove from her purse any pill bottles, as well as anything else that made her feel safe. "I will do the exposure without any safety net," she thought.
Sully went to the mall for about an hour. He was scared about doing the exposure at first, but 20 minutes after he got there his fear started to come down. He figured that if he started to feel panicky or if anything bad happened, he could just pop a pill.	Sally went to the mall for about 1 hour. Although she felt very anxious at first and wanted to leave, her anxiety came down within 15 minutes. She began to recognize that malls aren't really dangerous places. She became a bit bored with just walking around the mall and found herself going into a few stores.

It might seem that Sully and Sally both had successful exposure sessions. Both went to the mall for an hour, both experienced a decline in their anxiety, and neither had a full panic attack. But what lesson was each learning about the dangerousness of malls? Sally taught herself that the mall isn't a threat. She expected something bad might happen, but it didn't. Sully, on the other hand, taught himself that he can go to the mall if he takes along his medication in case he has a panic attack. Do you see how Sully still believes that malls could be dangerous, especially if he doesn't have his medication with him?

Look back at your self-assessment from Chapter 2 (Form 2.6 on page 50). What safety behaviors did you list? Since reading more about anxiety, exposure, and safety behaviors, can you add any other safety behaviors to the list? Record your responses on Form 8.4.

My Safety Behaviors

Anxiety problem	Safety behaviors
1.	
2.	
3.	

Safety Thoughts

In addition to enacting certain behaviors or carrying around safety objects, some anxious individuals develop safety thoughts or mental rituals that help them feel safer. These may include:

- Distracting yourself to force worrisome thoughts out of your mind
- Repeating phrases, mantras, or prayers over and over in your head
- Replacing unpleasant thoughts or images with "safe" thoughts or images

Use Form 8.5 to list any safety thoughts you can think of that you use when you're anxious.

Reducing Safety Behaviors and Thoughts

Since this book is all about helping you feel less anxious, why would we ask you to stop doing things that help you feel less anxious? As we mentioned, safety behaviors may help in the short term, but in the long run they make your anxiety stronger. All the thought-challenging and exposure exercises you are practicing are designed to help your brain *relearn* that the situations you fear are generally safe. Safety behaviors can block that from happening. Take a look at the normal chain of thoughts that happen when people do exposures:

I am afraid of *X* and think it is dangerous.
↓
I did exposures to *X*.
↓
I expected bad things to happen.
↓
Nothing bad happened.
↓
Therefore, maybe *X* isn't dangerous.
↓
X is actually safe.

Now see how safety behaviors interfere with this chain of thoughts:

I am afraid of *X* and think it is dangerous.
↓
I did exposures to *X,* but also used safety behaviors.
↓
I expected bad things to happen.
↓
Nothing bad happened because I used my safety behaviors.
↓
Something bad might have happened if I hadn't used the safety behaviors.
↓
X is still not safe.

My Safety Thoughts

Anxiety problem	Safety thoughts
1.	
2.	
3.	

What all this means is that as you increase your exposures, you need to decrease (and eventually eliminate) your use of safety behaviors. Some find it best to give them all up at once, but if that sounds too difficult, you can give them up more gradually.

For example, Maria had severe panic disorder and was terribly afraid to go outside her home. She could go out only when she was with her husband. When she started her exposures, she went outside for a walk around the block with her husband beside her. The next time, she went out with her husband trailing 50 yards behind her. The third time, she went around the block while her husband stayed home but talked to her on the cell phone the whole time. The fourth time, he wasn't on the phone, but they both had their phones ready in case she needed to call. By the fifth time, Maria went around the block by herself without her phone.

Stopping your safety behaviors all at once is often best, if possible. Next best is to reduce them as quickly as you can. Safety behaviors will only serve to help your anxiety thrive.

Troubleshooting

Throughout our many years of working with people who have problems with anxiety, we have seen virtually every problem that can creep in and get in the way of doing exposure. Below are some of the common issues, and some suggestions for how to overcome them.

Lack of time. Probably the most common difficulty we hear from our patients is that they believe they don't have the time to do exposures. This is understandable, as many of us lead busy lives and have many commitments. But you also need to make sure you schedule time for yourself. Think of it this way: anxiety eats up far too much of your time already, so try to give just as much time to overcoming your anxiety. In the long run, you'll find that a life free of anxiety gives you more free time, since you won't be wasting time with fears, worries, compulsions, or avoidance.

Lack of money or resources. We recognize that some, albeit certainly not all, exposures may have some financial costs. If your exposure involves making dinner for friends, groceries cost money. Exposures involving driving require gasoline. Going to some crowded places like movie theaters requires you to buy tickets. In some cases you can try to think of ways to minimize the costs, like going to a matinee or one of those theaters where they show older movies. Other times, unfortunately, there isn't much you can do about the cost. But think of this as an investment. Will you be more productive at work if you can overcome your fears? Would you be better able to get a promotion if you were anxiety-free? Could you go back to school and further your education after defeating your worries? Would you save money if you and your physician were able to reduce or eliminate your need for anxiety medication? A small investment now can have big returns later.

Lack of support from others. This can be a hard one. Occasionally people's families or friends are not very supportive of their attempts at self-improvement. This may be due to their own fears that you might change or that you won't need them anymore. It might be due to their own busy schedules that leave them little time, for example, to look after the children while you work on exposures. In some cases, family members may have become such a part of your anxiety routines that they become scared about what will happen to you if you try to confront your fears. Change, even positive change, can be difficult for some people. For example, a man may start to feel a bit insecure if after 15 years of being around all the time because she was afraid to leave her home, his wife suddenly feels comfortable going out with friends and isn't around as much. Parents, spouses, and other family members can start to feel they're no longer needed as their anxious loved ones become able to do more on their own. The best solution to problems of support is *communication*. Explain to your loved ones what you are doing, why you are doing it, and why it is important to you. Then listen to and discuss their worries or concerns. Most often, a lack of support is due to a misunderstanding about what will happen, which can be resolved through open and honest communication. If it can't, see if you can find support from someone else—a friend who can look after the children for an hour, a coworker who can cover for you while you do some quick exposures, a relative who can drive you to places you need to go for your exposure, or a therapist who can help support you emotionally through the process. Feel free to review the recommendations for friends and families in Chapter 3 and in the box below.

Tips for Family Members

- Ask how you can help. Be understanding if the best way to help is by *not* helping.

- Learn about your loved one's anxiety problem and its treatment.

- Try to see the anxiety from your loved one's perspective and be gentle if recovery takes time or has setbacks.

- Support the decision to work on overcoming anxiety.

- Be supportive rather than critical or controlling.

- Discuss how you can stop accommodating your loved one's fears.

- Communicate effectively and lovingly.

Fears that exposure will make things worse. This is a very common concern. In fact, a survey several years ago found that some mental health workers worry about this, too. But it is simply not true. When done properly, as we have described in this and the next three chapters, exposure is completely safe and will lead to a reduction in your fears in the long run. Of course it will feel scary—you are confronting your fears, after all!—but it isn't dangerous. It is like lifting weights. At first the weights feel too heavy and lifting them can be strenuous. But done properly, you will get stronger and the weight will be easier to lift. Eventually you will be able to move up to heavier weights, and the process will repeat. The same principles are at work with exposure. Done properly, you will be better and better able to manage each exposure, until you are able to move up to more difficult ones.

Conclusion

This chapter set the stage for you to begin the most powerful part of treatment—exposure. You learned several important steps:

1. You learned how exposure works and you developed an Exposure Plan.

   ■ The Exposure Plan listed your fears in order of difficulty.

   ■ You then rated each fear on a 0–100 scale to show how much anxiety each item on the list would probably cause you.

2. You learned how to set up an exposure practice.

   ■ You choose a practice that will be challenging but feasible.

   ■ You arrange the details of the practice.

   ■ You review your anxious thoughts.

   ■ You set clear and specific goals that focus on actions rather than feelings.

3. You learned about staying in the exposure situation until your fear comes down or you learn that your feared predictions are not true.

4. You learned to repeat the exposure until it no longer causes significant fear.

5. You discovered the importance of frequency, duration, and variety of exposures—why you should do many exposures over as long a period of time and in as many different circumstances as possible.

6. Finally, you learned about safety behaviors, why they are a problem, and the importance of eliminating them.

The following chapters will give you specific information about how to do different types of exposures. Chapter 9 outlines how to set up exposures to objects and situations. Chapter 10 discusses how to set up exposure to anxiety-provoking thoughts, images, or memories. Finally, Chapter 11 describes how to set up exposures to feared sensations in your body.

9

confronting feared objects and situations

If your Exposure Plan included facing feared objects or situations (as opposed to feared internal experiences, such as thoughts, feelings, and physical symptoms), this chapter will teach you strategies for overcoming exaggerated fears of virtually anything that is outside your body, including (but certainly not limited to):

- **Objects and animals:** animals and insects, blood, needles, exposure to germs (for example, being near sick people), exposure to chemicals (for example, bleach, gasoline)
- **Places and situations:** elevators, crowds, long lines, leaving the house alone, public transportation, enclosed spaces, open spaces, heights, storms, driving, flying, being out at night, being alone in a parking garage
- **Activities:** walking around the neighborhood, exercising, public speaking, dating, conversations, meeting new people, speaking up in meetings, interviews

Conducting Exposures to External Objects

People can develop fears of virtually any object, whether animal, vegetable, or mineral.

People can develop fears and phobias related to nearly every imaginable external object, including animal, vegetable, or mineral, and just about anything else on the planet. In many cases, fears are associated with objects that may be dangerous under certain circumstances, yet the fear extends to circumstances where the risk is small. For example, although cats can sometimes become aggressive, most of the time they are relatively safe when approached with care.

In other cases, people may fear objects that are virtually never dangerous. We have seen individuals who fear worms, cotton balls, things that are green in color, looking out the window of a tall building, or touching a photo of a spider or other animal. The general process of exposure remains the same regardless of the feared object. Tips for planning exposures for some of the more common fears are presented in the following sections.

Exposures to objects are usually easy to arrange, although you may need to be creative. Virtually any object can become associated with a fear, although some are more common than others. People have reported fears of certain weapons (whether or not a weapon has ever been used against them), machines, needles or syringes, certain words or numbers, and balloons. Most exposures to objects are straightforward to arrange. Animal fears are also quite common, but exposures to animals can be more difficult to arrange; with the exception of common household pets, most animals live in the wild and may not show up just when we need them! Some animals may be fairly rare in your area, requiring you to visit a zoo, exotic pet store, or other collection of animals. For some people, playing with fake or toy animals (like a rubber snake) or even looking at pictures or video clips of the feared animal is enough to arouse fear. This is particularly true for people who fear spiders, snakes, and insects.

Please use caution when practicing exposure with animals. If you're confronting your fear of dogs, for example, be sure you know something about the animal (for example, consider using a friend's pet) rather than getting close to a stray dog. Although it's usually safe to touch and hold certain animals with appropriate caution (such as ants, dogs, birds, harmless spiders), you should avoid handling animals that can cause harm, such as bees and wasps or unfamiliar spiders.

The box below through page 154 gives examples of where to find commonly feared objects and animals.

Locating Objects for Exposures

Blood

First of all, do not cut yourself for an exposure. If you are planning to do an exposure involving seeing blood or having your own blood drawn, you can make arrangements with a local blood donation center. They have professional phlebotomists (people who are trained to draw and handle blood) who can ensure that everything is done safely, cleanly, and properly. If you go at a time when they are not busy, the staff may also be willing to let you see anywhere from a drop of blood to a full bag of donated blood. Finally, the staff would likely be able to answer any questions you have.

Cats, dogs, and birds

Often, people with phobias of common household pets, such as dogs, cats, and birds, choose to practice exposure to the pets of their friends and family members. Other sources of these animals include pet stores and local parks or beaches where people walk their dogs, or you might see a bird in the wild. An animal shelter is also a good place to check. They often have kittens, puppies, and adult cats and dogs waiting to be adopted. If you ask, they may let you hold a cat or dog. (Watch out, though: they may try to convince you to adopt the animals!) If you choose to use a friend's cat or dog, you could start with your friend holding the animal while sitting on the other side of the room and then gradually work up to petting and holding the animal yourself. For dogs, you might want to try smaller dogs, such as Chihuahuas or

Pomeranians, at first and then work up to larger breeds like Labradors and golden retrievers. It is true that some animals might bite or scratch. Just ask your friends if their pets are ever aggressive. Approaching or holding unknown animals outdoors is *not* recommended.

Dirty or contaminated objects

Fears of contamination are very common. Fortunately, exposures to dirt or contamination are easy to set up. This is because for people with contamination fears, virtually everything may *seem* contaminated. Various places that can be used for exposures include kitchen counters, carpets or floors, dusty objects, toilets and bathroom fixtures, objects that have been outdoors, clothes that have not been washed, and so forth. The key to these exposures is to touch or hold the objects and then resist hand washing.

Locks, light switches, appliance switches, and the like

Most commonly, people develop these fears because they are concerned that they might not have properly locked the door, turned off the lights, or turned off an appliance and that something dangerous or bad will happen as a result. Exposures usually involve locking the door or flipping the switch once, leaving the area, and resisting the urge to go back to double check that the task was completed properly.

Needles and syringes

Pharmacies and medical practices regularly stock new clean and disinfected needles and syringes for a nominal cost. Used or discarded needles and syringes, or those that you cannot verify are clean, should not be handled. After conducting an exposure to needles or syringes, you should discard them in an appropriate "sharps container" like those found in many public restrooms, even if you have not broken the skin or drawn blood.

Mice and rodents

The best source for mice and rats is often your local pet store. Other possible sources include zoos or the biology or psychology department at your local university.

Snakes

Finding snakes for exposures can be difficult since they usually hide when people are around. For early exposures, many people find plastic or rubber snakes (like those found in toy stores) to be enough to make them anxious. Most zoos have snake pens for viewing. If you call ahead and explain your situation, the zoo staff may even join you and tell you about the snakes. If you are very lucky, the zoo's professional snake handler may even let you hold a nonpoisonous snake! We have also had success in pet stores that sell snakes. On several occasions, sales clerks have been willing to stay after the store closes (for a reasonable hourly rate) and work with an individual who fears snakes. Because some snakes are poisonous or aggressive, doing exposures by handling wild snakes found in nature is *not* recommended.

Spiders and insects (for example, bees, wasps, cockroaches, moths)

It may not be uncommon to see spiders and insects outdoors or even in your home, but finding them can be a challenge when you're actually looking for them. Also, if you fear spiders or insects, you may need to ask someone else to catch them for you. Depending on the types of bugs you fear, possible sources include your backyard, garden and plant stores, zoos, university biology departments, beekeepers, exterminators, and natural science museums. You can even order certain specimens through companies that sell biological supplies to schools and researchers (check out *www.carolina.com*). Pictures and videos (check out YouTube) can be helpful, too.

Storms

Of all the possible fears, storms are the one over which we have the least control. It's obviously impossible to ensure that a storm will come along just when you're ready for an exposure practice! Fortunately, weather forecasts are usually accurate enough that you can make sure you're ready for an exposure when a storm comes. When it does occur, make sure you look out the window, step out on your porch, and avoid safety behaviors such as compulsively checking weather forecasts or hiding in the basement. Some people find it helpful to start by listening to sounds of thunderstorms and imagining they're real. In addition, some practitioners may be able to treat storm phobias using virtual reality (VR) exposures (for a list of VR practitioners, check out *www.virtuallybetter.com*).

Weapons

As you can probably imagine, because weapons are specifically designed to cause harm it is important to exercise caution when considering exposures involving knives or firearms. In fact, many countries or regions have very specific laws regarding who may legally possess certain weapons. If you consider it important to your recovery to conduct exposures to weapons—for example, a police officer who developed a fear of handguns after his weapon accidentally discharged—then it is strongly recommended that you contact an accredited weapons safety trainer (perhaps through a handgun safety course) to assist you and ensure proper and safe handling of the weapons.

Exposures to Places, Situations, and Activities

When a person has a fear of being in or around certain places or situations, exposure practices usually involve going to those places or situations. You can become anxious in these places or situations for a variety of reasons. You might be worried about what other people will think of you. You might feel trapped and unable to escape. Perhaps certain places or situations remind you of something terrible that happened to you, like an assault or an accident. You can also start with places or situations that are only somewhat similar to the place or situation, like driving on a suburban street instead of driving on the highway. Once you feel comfortable with the somewhat similar situation, you can move up to bigger streets and eventually the highway. The box on pages 155–157 has some examples of how you can plan exposure practices involving a range of activities.

As you develop your Exposure Plan, it will be important to think of ways to vary the intensity of your exposure to these places or situations so you can gradually increase the difficulty of your practices. If you fear being in a large, crowded shopping mall by yourself, you might start by visiting a smaller mall during a slow time, with a family member or friend. Over time, you can work your way up to more difficult exposures by visiting different and larger malls and by gradually doing more exposures alone (perhaps initially having your "safe person" waiting in the parking lot and available by cell phone).

Planning Exposures Involving Places, Situations, and Activities

Airplanes

Many people have flying fears, but unfortunately exposure to airplanes is becoming increasingly difficult. Safety regulations for airlines and airports limit who can go on or around airplanes without a ticket. Some airlines have special programs to help people with fears of flying, so it might be a good idea to contact airlines to check. Also, some regional airlines offer inexpensive fares for very short flights that you can take advantage of. Finally, there is evidence that computer-administered "virtual reality" (VR) treatments may be helpful for fears of flying. You can find out about practitioners who use VR exposure treatments at *www.virtuallybetter.com.*

Arenas, malls, stadiums, and theaters

Large, crowded buildings are common in most areas, but gaining access to them can be difficult without buying a ticket to an event. You may be able to get special permission to enter the building for free during a time when no event is scheduled, or you may be able to practice exposure at an inexpensive or free event. Vary the intensity of the exposure by going to smaller (for example, high school stadiums) or larger (for example, professional or college stadiums) locations. You can also vary the intensity by going during less or more busy times (weekday matinee versus Saturday evening movie) or to less or more popular or busy events (a small symphony performance versus a large rock concert).

Assertiveness

Many people feel anxious when they need to be assertive. Sometimes this means having trouble saying no to an unreasonable request. Other times it could involve asking others to change their behavior in some way or to do something for you. Assertiveness can easily be practiced with strangers. Examples include phoning a store and asking the clerk to look up the price of an item, or buying something and then returning it the next day.

Authority figures

Talking to authority figures often feels like a difficult exposure to plan because people frequently think that "bothering" the authority figure could get them into trouble. The fact of the matter is that many people talk to others in positions of authority every day without making trouble. Examples of exposures include calling the nonemergency phone at a police station (obviously, **do not call 911 to practice**) and asking how to file an accident report or register a new bicycle, calling a fire station to ask for directions, or going to a medical clinic and asking the doctor questions.

Crowds

Exposures to crowds are usually similar to exposures involving arenas, malls, stadiums, or theaters. Referring back to that section will be helpful. Other examples of crowded places in which to practice include supermarkets, large restaurants, amusement parks, buses or subways (during rush hour), crowded elevators, flea markets, conventions, trade shows, and busy city streets.

Dating

While one could go to a local coffee shop or bar and ask many people out on dates, that might be disrespectful or bothersome to others who don't want to be bothered by a stranger. It would probably be more appropriate to join a singles club or a speed dating service where others are more likely to be looking to date as well. Many of these clubs or services do charge a fee. Alternatively, you could ask a friend or family member to set you up with someone they know is single. Remember, the goal of the exposures is to practice becoming comfortable with dating or asking someone out on a date, not to immediately find "the one."

Disorganization and messiness

Fears relating to messes, or having things disorganized or out of order, are often seen in people with obsessive–compulsive disorder (OCD), although anyone can develop similar fears. Exposure to disorganization or messiness involves intentionally rearranging things or making small messes without cleaning them up. For exposures to arouse anxiety, some people need to continue looking at the mess until their anxiety comes down. Others just need to *know* that the mess exists, even if they leave the area. (*Note*: You should discuss this exposure with others living in the same house or apartment before beginning.)

Doctor or dentist offices, hospitals

Depending on your fears, you can vary the intensity of your exposure by going to a small office, a local clinic, a large medical/dental practice, or a major hospital complex. Exposures to medical or dental offices are often fairly easy to set up. Because dentists, doctors, and nurses are health professionals, they may be willing to help you with your exposure practices.

Driving on city streets or highways

There are only a few places left that are not crisscrossed with highways or streets, so finding them is fairly easy. If the amount of traffic is a factor in your fear, start with exposures on less busy roads. For highway exposures, you may want to start with highways that have many on- and off-ramps so that you can build up from staying on the highway for just one exit to staying on for many exits. As you become more comfortable with smaller roads or deserted highways, you can start moving up to major freeways or interstate highways.

Specific people

It's common to develop fears relating to specific people or types of people after a traumatic event. For example, if a woman is raped, she will very commonly feel fearful around men for a while. If you were mugged or assaulted, it would not be unusual to become anxious or fearful around people who remind you of the attacker. Exposures might begin with interacting with people who remind you a bit of the person or people you fear, and then gradually interacting with people who are more and more like the specific person or people you fear. (*Note*: If someone committed a traumatic offense against you, your Exposure Plan should obviously *not* involve that person. No exposure practices should ever involve doing anything that most people would consider dangerous.)

Exercise or sports

You may be surprised to know that many people are fearful of exercising for a range of reasons. Some people, particularly those who have panic attacks, may be fearful of the physical sensations of panting or raising their heart rate. Some people may be anxious about sweating for social reasons or due to feelings of uncleanliness. Others may fear injury from exercise. And finally, some people may avoid exercise or sports because they think their performance will be judged. Think carefully about what it is that concerns you about exercising or playing sports and try to think of activities that you could do. Jogging or running is free. Most cities have gyms that you could join. For a fee, many cities have recreational programs where you could play basketball or tennis, or join hiking groups. If you have concerns about medical problems or your physical ability to engage in such activities, please check with your physician.

Heights, bridges

Exposure to heights can be fairly easy and safe to plan. Depending on the severity of your fear, initial exposures might involve standing on a stepladder, stool, or chair; on the balcony of a high-rise apartment; or near the window of a tall office building. Some larger buildings, such as the Empire State Building, have public observation decks that you may be able to use for practices. Bridges can be used as well, ranging from small concrete bridges to large steel and cable bridges located over large bodies of water. In some places, particularly mountainous areas, suspension bridges may even be a possibility.

Speeches

Fear of public speaking is one of the most common fears of all. Fortunately, there are many individuals, groups, and organizations that help people become more comfortable in front of an audience. One of the biggest (and least expensive) is Toastmasters International, which has chapters in many cities and towns around the world (see *www.toastmasters.org*). Groups meet regularly to practice giving speeches. The members can range from people with full-blown social phobia to experienced public figures. For less intense initial exposures, practice in front of a mirror, give a small speech while sitting in front of one or two friends, stand and deliver a speech to a few friends, or even stand up and say a few words at a formal occasion like a wedding.

Finally, many people develop fears of doing certain activities. Sometimes these are social activities, like public speaking or asking someone out on a date. The advantage of exposures with people is that you can start by asking someone you feel comfortable with to pretend to be someone who makes you anxious or roleplay the specific activity. The box on pages 155–157 has some examples of how you can plan to practice exposure involving particular activities in addition to those involving other people.

After You Identify and Plan Your Exposures

After you identify and plan your exposures, review the steps we described in Chapter 8. After deciding to practice exposures to feared objects, places, situations, or activities (based on your Exposure Plan), you will:

1. Plan the details of how you will find and confront the object, place, situation, or activity.

2. Identify the thoughts you're likely to experience during the exposure.

3. Set specific measurable goals based on actions, not feelings.

4. Start and stay in the exposure until your anxiety comes down.

5. Not use any safety behaviors or safety thoughts.

6. Finish the exposure, review your goals, and decide whether any of your anxiety-provoking thoughts or expectations came true.

7. Reward yourself for facing your fears.

Examples of Exposure Plans

Exposure Plans are very individual, so there's no such thing as a typical Exposure Plan. This section provides some examples of other people's Exposure Plans for fears that concern objects or situations, including the Exposure Plans for Bindi and Jacqui (both of whom you met in the Introduction to this book), as well as three other individuals—Miguel, Sandra, and Sunil. Don't think that your plan needs to look exactly like any of these, even if the person described in the example sounds a lot like you.

Bindi: Social Anxieties

You may remember Bindi from earlier in the book. She was the university student from a small rural town who became very anxious when she needed to talk to people or go to events like parties. Sample Completed Form 8.3 (Bindi) shows her Exposure Plan.

Bindi initially found developing the Exposure Plan to be a bit overwhelming, as she could come up with hundreds of situations that would make her anxious. As she worked through it, she simplified the process by focusing on either situations that were a frequent problem, like talking to classmates or giving presentations in class, or things that she really wanted to start doing, like going to parties or social gatherings.

Bindi started her exposure with item 10. Talking to classmates was easy enough to practice since most of her classes had a lot of students, and it was a situation over which she had a lot of control. She decided that she would talk to two different classmates every day. She felt that she could start by talking about the class—like asking questions about an upcoming assignment or how the other students liked the class. Bindi got very anxious the first time she did her exposure, with her fear rating going up to 80 (she had predicted it would be only 60), but her fear went down quickly. The classmate she talked to before class was quite friendly, and Bindi found out that her classmate was also from a rural community. She did her second exposure after class, talking to a young man who sat next to her during the lecture. This time her anxiety only went up to a 50. The conversation was also quite easy and her anxiety went down quickly again. Bindi thought he might have been "hitting" on her, but she felt like she wasn't ready to start thinking about dating or working on flirting yet. On the second and third days, her fear when talking to classmates never went above 15, so Bindi decided it was time to start a more challenging exposure. She moved up to #8 on her Exposure Plan, asking or answering a question at least once in each of her classes. Talking in class was more difficult than chatting with classmates because Bindi felt that she might give the wrong answer or ask a stupid question. Her fear rating started around 80, even though she expected it would be a 70 when she filled in her Exposure Plan. After a week of doing this exposure during every class, her anxiety rating never

Exposure Plan in Order of Difficulty

Rank order	Fear trigger: Situation, object, thought, or sensations	Fear rating (0–100)
1	Going out to a hip club	100
2	Going to a party where I don't know anyone	99
3	Going on a date	95
4	Going to a party where I know some people	85
5	Going out to a fancy restaurant with someone I know	84
6	Doing a presentation in one of my classes	80
7	Asking my professor questions during office hours	75
8	Talking/answering a question in class	70
9	Going out to a casual restaurant with someone I know	65
10	Talking to a classmate before or after class	60

got above 30 when speaking up in class. She said that she realized that "people ask questions in class all the time. It's the professor's job to answer the questions!"

Her next exposures to going out with others were difficult to plan. Bindi knew that she would find it easier to start by going out with people she knew, but the problem was that she didn't know many people very well at her university. So she modified her first exposure—talking to classmates—to ask them if they wanted to go and get coffee or a meal after class. She didn't ask the flirty guy, but the woman who was also from a rural town (Lynn) was really excited to grab dinner later that week. Apparently, Lynn didn't have many friends in the city either! They met for dinner at a bar and grill just off campus, and while Bindi really didn't feel like she "fit in" with the crowd there, she and Lynn had a nice time getting to know each other and laughing about how different life is in the city than in the country.

Bindi and Lynn began sitting beside each other in class and started to become good friends. Bindi felt comfortable enough to tell Lynn that she was working on meeting more people and "being less introverted," so Lynn invited Bindi to a book club gathering at her apartment. Bindi thought this would be a good way to start working on #4 on her Exposure Plan. This made her quite anxious, with a fear rating of 70, but it was actually easier than what she had expected. She also joined the university's Indigenous Students' Association so that she could meet more people, and possibly even start attending some of their social gatherings in the evenings (#2 on her Exposure Plan). She also heard that sometimes professors would ask the Indigenous Students' Association to give a classroom presentation on various aspects of their culture and history—a great way to practice #6 on her Exposure Plan.

Over the next few weeks, Bindi participated in a few of the classroom presentations, where her anxiety went up to a 60 but came down quickly when she saw how interested the class looked. She also went to a party with Lynn, which surprisingly wasn't too anxiety provoking, and she got to meet a few new people who she found interesting. She also decided to ask the flirty classmate from her second exposure if he wanted to get a coffee after class, as she thought this might be a good way to start practicing #3 on her Exposure Plan. She was a little disappointed when he said he already had plans with his boyfriend—apparently he wasn't flirting after all—but she realized that talking to him and asking him out still counted as an exposure. As fate would have it, though, the next week a guy she had met at an Indigenous Students' Association social event asked her out for a drink in the city. Bindi was a little terrified, because this was both #3 and possibly #1 on her Exposure Plan, but she was feeling buoyed by the success she had been having with her previous exposures. The date was a little awkward because they didn't have a lot in common, and the place they went to wasn't exactly a "hip club," but Bindi felt that it still counted as a successful exposure. Her anxiety went up to a 70 at first but, as with her previous exposures, it came down fairly quickly. During the date, the guy mentioned that he had been to a new local hot spot recently, so a couple of days later Bindi suggested to Lynn that they should get dressed up on Friday night and check it out.

Since that time, Bindi has taken every opportunity to talk to more people and get out of her dorm room as much as possible. Because of her studies and the fact that finances are tight as a student, she goes out to dinner or clubs only once every 2 or 3 weeks. Even so, she has realized how much more comfortable she is when she does go out. She still feels a little anxious at times in new situations or when meeting new people, but she keeps pushing herself because she knows that she can beat her anxiety and live life the way she wants.

Jacqui: Thoughts of Harm

In Chapter 8, you reviewed the Exposure Plan for Jacqui, the new mother who had been having intrusive thoughts about harming her new daughter. Take a look at Jacqui's Exposure Plan in Sample Completed Form 8.3 (Jacqui), repeated here, to remind yourself of her triggers and her plans for exposure. Her Exposure Plan focused on two types of things—the intrusive thoughts, which will be discussed in Chapter 10, and situations or objects that seem to cause those thoughts to pop into her mind. We'll discuss her exposures to the situations and objects here.

While looking over her Exposure Plan, Jacqui noticed that many of the items listed fell into two categories: (1) situations where *she* thinks she might actually cause harm to her child (driving with her child, objects that could possibly be used to harm the infant) and (2) situations where *others* might think she has harmed or neglected her child. Given that the items about what others might think were rated as less anxiety provoking, Jacqui decided to start with those. She decided to book an appointment with her daughter's pediatrician for a checkup but asked her partner to drive them to the medical office since she wasn't ready to drive with her daughter alone. The night before the appointment, Jacqui was so anxious that she couldn't sleep and spent much of the night ruminating about all of the things that could go wrong. Not surprisingly, when they arrived at the pediatrician's office the next day, Jacqui's anxiety was through the roof. On her Exposure Plan she thought it would only go up to an anxiety rating of 40 out of 100, but once she went into the waiting room, it was closer to 80 out of 100. She desperately wanted to cancel the appointment and leave, but she had an even stronger desire to overcome her anxiety for the sake of her daughter. "I don't want her to grow up seeing her mother like this," she thought. So she stayed.

Despite Jacqui's worst expectations, the appointment went just fine. Her daughter was completely healthy, although the pediatrician did say that her daughter's weight was a little lower than expected for her age. Hearing this, Jacqui became worried that this meant she was a bad mother and was somehow neglecting her child's health, but the pediatrician reassured her that some babies have periods of time when their weight gain simply slows down. Jacqui was very relieved to hear the pediatrician say, "It looks like you're doing everything right as a new mother." By the end of the appointment, Jacqui's anxiety had gone down from the 80 in the waiting room to a 20.

Given her success in facing #10 on her Exposure Plan, Jacqui decided to move up to #8 and ask her in-laws if they would babysit her daughter for an hour two times during the week. Jacqui's mother-in-law was ecstatic about getting to spend extra time with her granddaughter and even offered to babysit more often than twice per week. Jacqui was tempted by the offer but decided to stick with her initial Exposure Plan for a few weeks and then she would increase the number of visits. The next day, Jacqui put her daughter in the stroller, and they walked over to her mother-in-law's house for their visit. Jacqui decided that she would spend the hour at the nearby shopping center. As she walked to the shops, Jacqui became very anxious that her mother-in-law might be noticing marks or bruises on her daughter and calling child protective services. Her anxiety went up to a 60 and, despite knowing that she should not engage in any safety behaviors, she called her mother-in-law to "make sure everything is okay." Her mother-in-law just laughed, said that everything was wonderful, and told Jacqui to enjoy her free time. Initially, this reassured Jacqui, but after about 15 minutes she started to worry again. This time

Exposure Plan in Order of Difficulty

Rank order	Fear trigger: Situation, object, thought, or sensations	Fear rating (0–100)
1	Having anything around that could potentially be a weapon (like a pencil) when I'm alone with my daughter	90
2	Changing my daughter's diaper when alone	85
3	Having thoughts that I might have poisoned my daughter	85
4	Having thoughts that I might have touched my daughter	80
5	Changing my daughter's diaper when my partner is around	80
6	Driving on the freeway with daughter	60
7	Hearing my daughter cry at night—worry I did something wrong	50
8	Dropping my daughter off at my in-laws'—worry they will find something that looks like an injury	50
9	Driving in my car on regular streets with daughter	40
10	Taking daughter to physician — worry she will find something that looks like an injury	40

she resisted the temptation to check again and continued doing some shopping. After about 30 more minutes, Jacqui was surprised to notice that her anxiety had gone down to about a 40; by the time her phone reminded her to walk back to pick up her daughter, her anxiety had gone down to a 15! And when she got back to her mother-in-law's house, there was no sign that any of her concerns had come true. The two of them had a delightful visit, and now her daughter was happily taking a nap.

Two days later, Jacqui dropped her daughter off again and went to the grocery store. This time her anxiety only went up to a 30, and she only had mild transient thoughts that her mother-in-law might find marks or bruises. So Jacqui decided that next time she would increase the difficulty of her exposure by driving her daughter the short distance to and from her mother-in-law's house. Not only would that let her start working on #9 on her Exposure Plan but also, if she drove she could use the car to go to see a movie. When she did drive her daughter over for the visit, she had a few thoughts like "What if I cause an accident and hurt my baby?" and "I might have left my daughter in the car seat bassinet on the driveway," which sent her anxiety up to a 40, but the drive there and back was uneventful. Each time she practiced this exposure over the next 2 weeks, it got easier and easier, and her anxiety never went above 20. Plus, she finally got to see several movies that her partner had no interest in watching! During the next several months, Jacqui kept pushing herself up through her Exposure Plan. Since she was enjoying going to the movies, she decided to take her daughter to an animated kid's movie, which required Jacqui to drive on the highway. Given how well these exposures were going, she decided it was time to shift her attention to doing exposures to her intrusive thoughts about harming or poisoning her daughter. But you'll have to read Chapter 10 to find out how well that went.

Miguel: Agoraphobia

Miguel is a 35-year-old man who experiences severe anxiety and panic attacks when he is in crowded places. Miguel becomes very anxious and panicky when he feels trapped or unable to escape from these places. Sample Completed Form 8.3 (Miguel) is a copy of Miguel's Exposure Plan.

Miguel started his exposure with item 10. Going to the supermarket in the evening was easy enough to practice, and it was a situation over which he had a lot of control. He decided that he would split up his shopping list into three parts and go around 8:30 P.M. on Monday, Wednesday, and Thursday. Miguel had a fear rating of 50 (he had predicted it would be only 30) before the first shop on the first day, but his fear went down quickly. On the second and third days, his fear about going to the supermarket on weekday evenings never went above 15. Miguel decided it was time to start a more challenging exposure. He moved up to going to the supermarket during busy times, such as Friday evening and weekend mornings, and decided to go to a different and bigger supermarket.

Shopping for groceries at busy times was more difficult than weekday evenings, and his fear rating started around 70, even though his expected fear rating on the Exposure Plan was a 55. After 3 days of this exposure, his anxiety rating never got above 30 when going to any supermarket at any time. Public transportation, whether buses, trains, or subways, was also difficult to get going. Miguel realized that he wasn't just nervous about being trapped, but he also feared

Exposure Plan in Order of Difficulty

Rank order	Fear trigger: Situation, object, thought, or sensations	Fear rating (0–100)
1	Going to the big mall around Christmas	100
2	Going to concerts or sports in big arenas	95
3	Going to the big mall on weekends.	90
4	Crowded movie theaters and being stuck in the middle of a row	80
5	Going to the mall on weekday nights	70
6	Subways or city trains – can't get off until the next stop	60
7	Going to the supermarket at busy times (weekend mornings)	55
8	Crowded buses – easier than trains because next stop usually closer	50
9	Crowded elevators	40
10	Going to the supermarket late in the evening on a weeknight (when there's only a few people there)	30

that he would have a panic attack and everyone would think he was crazy or weird. So he modified his plan and decided to take the bus at times when there would be fewer people riding it.

The following week he decided to tackle going to the mall. Christmas was 2 months away, and he wanted to start early so that he could build up to the top of his Exposure Plan. He went to the mall on a weekday evening. He was surprised at how busy it was—he assumed only a few people would be there—and he didn't end up going in. His anxiety hit about 85. After going home, Miguel was disappointed in himself, but realized that his anxiety went higher than expected because he was shocked by the number of people there.

The next day, Miguel returned to the mall more determined and more prepared for the number of people who would be there. And even though there were almost as many people in the mall as there had been the night before, Miguel went in and browsed the shops for an hour. His fear rating only went up to 60 this time and came down quickly to 25, although it briefly went back up to 50 when he went into the food court and saw a huge number of teenagers hanging out.

Over the next 3 weeks, Miguel started going to the malls on weekends and occasionally started taking public transportation to get there. He also started branching out to other malls, including one he could take the train to. He also decided to start watching movies at the theater in the mall.

He felt quite anxious about going to a movie, because he had the thought that if he had a panic attack and had to run out of the theater, he would still be in the crowded mall and would need to run out of there too. But he was comforted by the knowledge that his previous exposures had been successful and he hadn't had a full panic attack during any of them. He worked on countering his anxiety-related thoughts by asking himself, "What is really the worst that could happen? Some teenagers might think I'm weird . . . and I could live with that. I don't really care what teenagers think of me." Miguel was a little disappointed with the movie—it was one of those silly holiday comedies—but to his surprise he did spend more time laughing than being anxious.

Bolstered by his success with malls and movie theaters, Miguel pushed toward the top of his Exposure Plan. If he could overcome the easier fears, he figured he could also overcome the more difficult ones, and he was thrilled to think that he would no longer be under the control of his anxiety. He knew that a popular band he really enjoyed was playing a concert at the arena the next week, and his favorite baseball team was about to start a four-game stretch of home games. The baseball schedule was kind to him; the first two games would be against weak teams so he didn't think as many people would be going. The last two games were against his team's archrivals, so he knew the stadium would be packed. As expected, the stadium was fairly empty during the first game, and Miguel didn't experience much anxiety at all, about 50 at most. During the second game the next night, the team was doing a bobblehead giveaway and there were many more people. But his anxiety still only went up to a 50, which Miguel believed was due to his having already done this exposure the night before. The next two games against the archrivals were nearly sold out, but again his anxiety only hit 50 during the first game and 40 during the second one. In fact, Miguel started to think about getting season tickets, but decided against it when he saw how much the tickets cost! Finally, he went to the concert. He bought a ticket for a seat that was pretty far from the stage, but this was mostly because at age 35 he really didn't feel any desire to be on the floor level with the kids. What's more, his anxiety never went above

30 during the whole concert, although it did briefly go up to 50 afterward, when the thousands of people in the arena were all leaving at the same time.

As Christmas was approaching, Miguel was feeling quite confident about going to the mall no matter how busy it got. He was quite enjoying being able to get gifts for his nieces and nephews, but he felt like he already got the best present for himself: freedom from his anxiety.

Sandra: Blood, Injuries, and Injections

Since childhood, Sandra has always had an intense fear of seeing blood or injuries, as well as getting blood drawn or needles. She has never passed out at the sight of blood, but she regularly gets lightheaded and queasy. She doesn't watch contact sports because she worries that there might be a severe injury. Although she wishes she could donate blood, she has never seriously considered doing so. In fact, she generally avoids going to the doctor because she worries that she will have to get a shot or have blood drawn. And when her elderly father was in the hospital recently for a procedure, Sandra was unable to visit him because of her fears that she would see blood, needles, and IVs. Take a look at Sandra's Exposure Plan in Sample Completed Form 8.3 (Sandra).

Sunil: Fear of Cats

Sunil's fears were more focused than the others. When he was 11 years old, he went over to a friend's house one evening. His friend's family had a large and beautiful cat that he wanted to play with. When he got near the cat, it turned toward him and the hairs on its back bristled. Then it let out a loud hiss and narrowly missed scratching him. Now, 10 years later, Sunil still gets very anxious whenever he is around a cat.

He has no idea why this event affected him so much. He now lives in an apartment complex and has a neighbor with an outdoor cat. If Sunil sees the cat sleeping near the entrance to his apartment, he feels embarrassed by the fact that he must walk around the building and go in the side entrance. Take a look at his Exposure Plan in Sample Completed Form 8.3 (Sunil).

Improving Relevant Skills

Sometimes a person's fear is compounded because he lacks certain basic skills that are required to be safe or competent in the situation. For example, some people who fear skiing may lack the experience and training to be able to ski safely. They may benefit from some skiing lessons in addition to standard exposure practices.

But before you decide that you lack certain skills, it's important to know that your skills are probably better than you think they are. Most people with anxiety disorders *think* they have poor skills, but many research studies have shown that when objective judges watch people with anxiety, the judges rate their skills and performance more positively than the individuals rate their own skills and performance. This has been shown for public speaking, driving, small-talk

Do I actually lack some skills, or am I just too anxious to use the skills?

Exposure Plan in Order of Difficulty

Rank order	Fear trigger: Situation, object, thought, or sensations	Fear rating (0–100)
1	Giving/donating blood	100
2	Seeing someone with a severe injury, like a car accident victim	100
3	Being in the emergency room	99.9
4	Being in the regular hospital	90
5	Having to get an IV line	85
6	Having a small cut that's bleeding	80
7	Watching hospital-type TV shows	75
8	Getting a flu shot	70
9	Seeing someone with a small cut that's bleeding	50
10	Seeing dried blood on the ground	30

Exposure Plan in Order of Difficulty

Rank order	Fear trigger: Situation, object, thought, or sensations	Fear rating (0–100)
1	Petting a large cat while it is sitting on my lap	80
2	Petting a cat that is on the ground	75
3	Being in the same room with a cat (not petting it)	60
4	Going to a friend's house with a cat in the room	50
5	Walking past my neighbor's cat	50
6	Going to a friend's house with a cat in another room	40
7	Walking into my apartment building if I don't see my neighbor's cat (it might be hiding)	40
8	Seeing cats on TV	30

conversation, and even sports. The main issue isn't with their skills or performance; it's with their thoughts about their skills or performance, just like you learned in Chapters 5–7. So before you decide that your fears are due to a lack of relevant skills, take a moment to practice evaluating and challenging these thoughts to see if they are exaggerated or actually realistic. If you still feel like you may lack certain skills, such as driving, social interactions or public speaking, or studying and test taking, the box on the facing page lists some suggestions and resources that may be helpful.

Suggestions and Recommendations for Improving Skills

Driving Skills

Most people who fear driving actually drive very well. Unlike confident drivers, they rarely speed and they hold the steering wheel with both hands. Nevertheless, there are some fearful drivers who *should* be afraid because they drive unsafely. Often, these fearful drivers have very little driving experience. An example might be someone who obtained a license as a teenager and then spent the next 20 years avoiding driving until finally deciding to overcome his fear. If you are fearful of driving and also lack basic driving skills, it can be useful to combine exposure practices with driving lessons from a certified driving instructor. If you can't find one on your own, the government agency that handles driver's licenses (in the United States, this is usually your state's department of motor vehicles, or DMV) might be able to provide some recommendations. Some driving instructors even specialize in training fearful drivers, which can be helpful because they are more likely to be supportive and understanding of the fear.

Social and Communication Skills

Most people with high levels of anxiety in social situations have fine social skills, though they may feel socially awkward from time to time. For some people, though, a lifetime of avoiding social situations may prevent them from mastering some of the subtleties of social interaction. Some of the skills that may be lacking include asking someone out on a date, basic presentation skills, using nonverbal communication and body language effectively, how to be assertive, strategies for dealing with disagreements and conflict, and so forth. A full discussion of strategies for improving social skills is beyond the scope of this book, though there are excellent books on this topic. Organizations like Toastmasters International are excellent for helping people develop public speaking skills.

Studying and Test-Taking Skills

Many people with test-related anxiety have perfectly good studying and test-taking skills. Despite experiencing significant anxiety about doing poorly on tests, they typically do much better than expected. However, for some people, test anxiety is a realistic concern. Their performance on tests and exams is not as strong as it might be, possibly because they haven't learned effective study habits or test-taking skills. Most universities, colleges, and schools have special programs and departments designed specifically for people who are having difficulty with studying and test taking. If you are an enrolled student, you can usually access these programs for free. Just contact Student Services at the school or university, and they can help you access the services. If you are not currently a student—perhaps you are thinking of going back to school—Student Services may be able to point you in the direction of local organizations that specialize in helping learners improve their skills. Finally, many universities have excellent online tips and strategies for studying and test taking that can be accessed by anyone, including the universities that we each work at (*www.monash.edu/rlo/study-skills/preparing-for-exams/exam-strategies* and *www.ryerson.ca/studentlearningsupport/online-resources*).

Troubleshooting

Of course, not everyone's Exposure Plan will go smoothly, although many do when an individual really makes a commitment to the plan. But sometimes an exposure may go in the wrong direction. Bindi asked a male classmate out on a date, but he said no because he is not romantically attracted to women. Miguel was caught off guard about how busy the mall was on a weekday evening and didn't do his exposure. Even the best public speakers mess up a speech at times (just watch politicians on TV!). Even the cleanest people get sick from a bug every now and then. A dog might bark at you. You might feel woozy when standing near the window in a tall building. In fact, it's best to *expect* that setbacks will happen once in a while during the process. Then you can prepare for them to make sure they don't derail your motivation.

Remember that the anxious mind can play tricks on itself. As discussed in Chapter 5, we often pay attention to things and remember information in a biased fashion. The anxious mind is incredibly good at remembering when things go wrong, but it forgets the dozens or hundreds of times when things go right. Be sure to remember the times when nothing bad happened! It's a useful way of ensuring that you evaluate the actual risk in situations as realistically as possible.

Don't just remember the one time you drove on the freeway and another driver cut you off; also remember the 20 times you drove on the freeway last month when absolutely nothing bad happened. Keep the situation in perspective. Remind yourself that "I only got cut off once in 20 times, and it was just a 'close call.' I didn't get into an accident, I didn't lose control of my car, and I certainly didn't die in a fiery crash like I expected." Then get back on board with your Exposure Plan. Prove to yourself that the negative event was just a fluke or a coincidence.

10

confronting scary thoughts, memories, images, urges, and uncertainty

This chapter provides help when you can't stop intrusive thoughts, worries, images, urges, or memories from triggering strong feelings of fear. Some common examples of frightening thoughts include:

- Memories of traumatic experiences that repeatedly jump back into your mind
- Repeated and unrealistic worries
- Flashbacks to a combat experience
- Strange or disturbing urges that keep coming to mind
- Recurring feelings that something bad might happen
- Fear of being uncertain of things

Having thoughts like these doesn't automatically mean you have a problem and need to start exposure therapy—everyone has thoughts like these from time to time. But if these types of thoughts *repeatedly* come into your mind, despite your best efforts not to think about them, and if they are frightening to you, the exercises in this chapter may be useful.

Examples of Common Feared Thoughts, Memories, Images, Urges, or Uncertainty

Feared thoughts can take the form of (1) memories of past events, (2) thoughts of bad things that might happen in the future, (3) thoughts about something happening right now, and (4) worries about uncertainty.

171

Memories of the Past

Having recurring painful memories of past events is extremely common in posttraumatic stress disorder (PTSD). Some examples include:

- Feeling like your car accident is happening again and again

- Repeated nightmares about the time you were assaulted

- Disturbing mental images from a mass shooting, a hurricane, or some other public catastrophe that won't go away

- Recurring frightening memories about your time in combat

People without PTSD can also have recurring upsetting memories even if the memories aren't of an event in which their lives were really in danger. For example, people with social fears may have repeated memories about the one time they really messed up when presenting a book report in class. A person with panic attacks might not be able to shake the memory of his first panic attack, when he was in a large supermarket and was sure he was dying of a heart attack.

Fears of the Future

Fears of the future usually take the form of "What if . . . ?" worries. Some common recurring worries include:

- "What if my spouse was in an accident on the way to work?"—even if there's no reason to suspect that happened

- "What if I run out of money?"—even though you have plenty of money in your bank accounts

- "What if I don't pass my college classes?"—even though you have received straight-A grades in all your classes

- "What if there's something medically wrong with me?"—even though your doctor keeps telling you that you're healthy

These worries are common in generalized anxiety disorder (GAD), although anyone— even people without an anxiety disorder—can be bothered by recurring worries. However, it is important to distinguish between excessive worries and legitimate worries. A legitimate worry might be worrying frequently about the health of a loved one who has recently been diagnosed with a malignant cancer, whereas an excessive worry might be worrying frequently about the health of a loved one who is perfectly healthy. Similarly, repeated worries about finances when you are in significant debt that you cannot pay would be legitimate, whereas repeated worries about finances when you have strong savings and no debt would likely be excessive.

Urges and Images in the Present

Bothersome thoughts in the present are those that just come to mind and upset you. They aren't memories of bad things that happened previously; nor are they really worries about something possibly happening in the future. They're just thoughts or urges that you don't want to have but that keep coming into your mind. Examples of these thoughts include:

- Upsetting sexual urges that go against your personal sexual morals
- Recurring disturbing images of a religious, sexual, or moral nature that come to mind
- Urges to scream and tear off your clothes in public, even though you would never do that
- Impulses to count things in a certain way
- Disturbing urges to say something inappropriate or to hurt a loved one, even though you wouldn't act on these urges

Fear of Uncertainty

The final type of bothersome thought is related to feelings of uncertainty, of not knowing for sure how things are going to turn out. While uncertainty is a part of most anxiety problems—if someone with a dog phobia knew *for certain* that a dog couldn't bite him, he probably wouldn't be as scared—some people seem to be particularly intolerant of any uncertainty regardless of the source. This seems to be why some people's anxiety is so generalized and they worry and become anxious about everything. Examples of uncertainty include:

- Not recommending a restaurant to friends in case they get food poisoning, unless you know for certain that the restaurant practices perfect food hygiene
- Not picking a movie to watch until you are convinced from all of the reviews that you'll like it
- Not going on a trip somewhere unless you know exactly where you will be staying and exactly what you will be doing
- Repeatedly seeking reassurance before making even minor decisions
- Not participating in activities without being 100% sure you know how to go about them properly

Conducting Exposure to Thoughts, Memories, Images, and Urges

If you read Chapter 8, you already know what's involved in confronting thoughts, memories, images, and urges. The steps involved here are exactly the same. After you decide, based on your Exposure Plan, that you're going to do exposures to thoughts, memories, images, and urges, you will:

1. Plan the details of how you'll find and confront the thoughts, memories, images, or urges

2. Identify the thoughts you're likely to experience during the exposure

3. Set specific measurable goals based on actions, not feelings

4. Start the exposure

5. Stay in the exposure until your anxiety decreases or you learn that your feared consequences don't occur

6. Refrain from using any safety behaviors or safety thoughts

7. Finish the exposure

8. Review your goals and assess whether any of your anxious thoughts or expectations came true

9. Reward yourself for facing your fears

Exposure involves intentionally thinking your scary thoughts instead of trying to avoid, suppress, or distract yourself as usual. You need to force yourself to think these thoughts, just as Joseph needed to force himself to repeatedly jump off the diving board in Chapter 8. With repeated exposure, your memories, thoughts, images, and urges will become less frightening and eventually less frequent.

Trying Not to Think about Something versus Not Thinking about It

Try this little exercise. Below is Spotty the Polar Bear. Spotty is normally a mild-mannered bear, but he gets *very* upset when people start thinking about him. You don't want to upset a polar bear, so cover the page and do whatever you can not to think about Spotty for 1 minute. No matter what, make sure that the image of Spotty does not enter your mind.

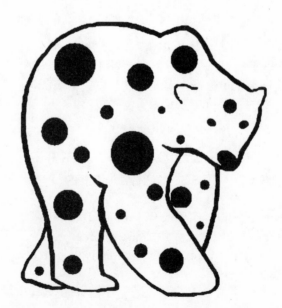

How did you do with this little exercise? Nearly everyone thinks about Spotty when they're trying not to. Why is it that when you're trying *not* to have a thought, you can't help having it?

The human brain is a wonderful machine, but it works in strange ways. Unlike our computers and smartphones, we don't have a "Delete" key or trash can icon that will get rid of things we don't want. Our brains are designed to think about things, in particular about important things. For some reason that scientists haven't quite figured out yet, when we try intentionally to forget or *not* think about something, our brains put the equivalent of a "VERY IMPORTANT" sticky note on that thought. And then our brains keep trying to think that "very important" thought!

Do I try to avoid unpleasant thoughts or memories?

It works the same way with disturbing thoughts or painful memories. The more we try not to dwell on them, the more likely it is that we will experience these intrusive thoughts or memories. In fact, the best way to ensure that your frightening thoughts or memories lose their "Very Important" label is to intentionally invite those thoughts or memories into your mind until they lose their power to frighten you.

You're not trying to turn bad thoughts into good thoughts or painful memories into happy memories. Rather, you want to get to the point where you can experience those thoughts without all the fear and negative emotions that go along with them. Let the thought become just a thought, rather than a thought that is perceived as dangerous or threatening.

For people with fears of external objects or situations, developing an Exposure Plan and carrying out specific exposures is a relatively straightforward activity. But people with fears of thoughts, memories, urges, and impulses often have a harder time. Three techniques can be very helpful:

1. People with either distressing memories of the past or scary worries about the future find it helpful to develop a worry/trauma exposure story.

2. People who have disturbing images or bothersome urges can benefit from forced-thought exposure practices.

3. People who are anxious about uncertainty can benefit from exposure to uncertainty.

We'll take you through the steps of how to develop each of these techniques.

Creating a Worry/Trauma Exposure Story

The goal of exposure to worries or memories is to experience those thoughts repeatedly until they stop carrying so much emotion with them. The exercise with Spotty showed you that trying *not* to think about those thoughts doesn't work. Instead, intentionally trying to invoke those thoughts gradually causes them to lose their power over you, in exactly the same way that a scary movie becomes less frightening if you watch it over and over and over.

Developing a worry/trauma script involves re-creating your memory over and over. Some of our former patients have opted to write out the memory like a movie script and then read it to themselves or out loud. Others have decided to narrate out loud and record the story using a voice recorder app on their phone or computer and then listen to it repeatedly. Neither approach is better or worse, so just pick what you would prefer. But do choose one of these types of options, as they create a permanent record that you can use repeatedly. We have found that when people try to make up the story anew each time—that is, just making it up each time they do an exposure—the quality of the story goes down. People end up skipping or avoiding some parts, or the story changes in little ways. When it is written down or recorded, you can be sure that you are doing the exact same exposure every time.

But either way you choose, be sure to include everything that happened (for memories) or everything you fear might happen (for worries)—the full story, from beginning to end. You don't need to do this all in one sitting, but you should devote at least an hour a day to preparing your story until it's complete. The keys to a worry/trauma story are:

- Write or speak it in the first person:
  - *"I walk down the hall"* instead of *"He walks down the hall."*
- Write or speak it in the present tense:
  - *"I walk down the hall"* instead of *"I walked down the hall."*
- Write or speak with detailed description and vivid images:
  - *"I can see his angry, pockmarked face as he reaches out and grabs me by the neck"* instead of *"The perpetrator proceeded to grasp me by the neck."*
- In addition to images, include all your senses:
  - *"I smell the formaldehyde as I push open the heavy creaking door into the morgue"* instead of *"I walk into the morgue."*
- Don't use words that soften the story:
  - *"The officer tells me that they're all dead"* instead of *"The officer tells me that they have all passed away."*

Most worry/trauma stories will take several attempts before they're just right and include all the details. You can start with rereading or rerecording early versions of your story. But after you've read or listened to it several times, add more details according to these guidelines and continue your practices by reading the new version several times.

While trauma scripts are an essential part of treatment (this is backed up by dozens of research studies and treatment guidelines), a small number of people who have experienced very traumatic events can become "overengaged" in their trauma scripts. They throw themselves into reliving the memory so clearly that they experience very severe anxiety or panic and sometimes dissociation. In dissociation your mind retreats from your own thoughts, feelings, and awareness of your surroundings. It isn't common and is only temporary, but if you do experience these feelings when going over your trauma script, you can take some simple tips to minimize them. The easiest ones are to change your script from present tense (which we recommended earlier) to past tense and to keep your eyes open while listening to the script. Both of these things will keep you a bit more grounded during the exposure. Once you are feeling more comfortable with the memories this way, you can start to move back to the present tense and closing your eyes.

If you have a lot of different worries, or if you have multiple disturbing memories, briefly describe them on your Exposure Plan form. Rate how much fear (on the 0–100 scale) it would cause you to read or listen to those scripts and then rank them from 1 (hardest) to 10 (easiest). Then, as in any other exposure, find the point on the Exposure Plan where you feel you can start. As you read or listen to your story, overcome the fears and allow the worries or memories to lose their power, you can move up to more distressing worry/trauma stories.

Pat: Different Worries, Different Scripts

Pat's Exposure Plan for worry stories is shown in Sample Completed Form 8.3, for Worry Scripts (Pat). Pat decided to list four different common worries and to use two different versions: one that is only moderately detailed (and therefore less frightening) and one that is very detailed (and therefore more frightening).

People commonly say, "I only have one traumatic memory, and it's the hardest item on my Exposure Plan. How do I find an easier memory to start with?" In this case, it's useful to develop several stories of varying difficulty by making each draft increasingly more detailed and graphic than the one before. Start with a version that is manageable. After reading or listening to it several times, you'll find that it becomes less frightening. Now develop another version, with more details.

Valerie: The Worst Fear

Now read Valerie's worry story. Valerie experiences frequent anxiety, where her mind creates all sorts of horrible worries, including worries about things that might have happened to her husband, Carl. In fact, she worries nearly every day about a whole range of things, including her health, her finances, and her marriage. Her worries about her marriage are particularly distressing, despite her knowledge that she and her husband have a wonderful relationship. Even so, she can't help worrying that suddenly her husband might find her unattractive and leave her.

Valerie felt uncomfortable keeping an audio version on her phone, and she hated how her recorded voice sounds, so she decided to write it out instead:

It's 3:00 on a Tuesday afternoon. My day at work seemed long because I couldn't concentrate due to my worries. I've tried to call Carl to check in and see if he is okay, but I keep getting his annoying voicemail message. I'm tired and stressed, so I decide to leave work early to head home and relax. I pull around the corner onto our street and immediately see Carl's truck as well as a red sports car in the driveway. I don't recognize the car, and I start to feel a nauseous feeling in my gut. I park on the street in front of the house and walk slowly up the driveway. As I pass by the red car, I look in and see a woman's stuff on the dashboard . . . a lipstick case and a hair scrunchy. My heart is pounding and I can almost taste my own vomit.

I walk to the front door and slowly, quietly slide my key into the lock. All of the blinds

Exposure Plan in Order of Difficulty

Rank order	Fear trigger: Situation, object, thought, or sensations	Fear rating (0–100)
1	Worrying about my girlfriend being killed in a car accident on the way to work (very detailed script)	100
2	Worrying about my parents' health or possible Alzheimer's disease (very detailed script)	90
3	Worrying about my girlfriend being killed in a car accident on the way to work (moderately detailed script)	85
4	Worrying that I don't have enough money to pay the rent and I'll get evicted (very detailed script)	80
5	Worrying that worrying so much will cause me to go crazy and get put in an asylum (very detailed script)	70
6	Worrying about my parents' health or possible Alzheimer's disease (moderately detailed script)	70
7	Worrying that I don't have enough money to pay the rent and I'll get evicted (moderately detailed script)	60
8	Worrying that worrying so much will cause me to go crazy and get put in an asylum (moderately detailed script)	50

are drawn, so I can't see in the windows. I slowly open the door and immediately smell a faint perfume. It's not mine. I hear my own heart pounding, but then I hear the muffled voices of Carl and a woman coming from the bedroom. I gingerly walk down the hall toward the bedroom and press my ear against the closed door. I still can't hear what they're saying, but I hear the woman giggling. I open the door a crack and peer in. Oh, my God. It's what I feared most. Carl is in bed with another woman. And she is so beautiful, not like me. As the tears stream down my face, I realize how unattractive I am. She's the type of beautiful woman that Carl deserves.

They both look up, hearing my pathetic sobs. And Carl doesn't even try to make excuses. Why should he? They both start laughing at me as I turn and run out of the house. I keep running down the street, ignoring my car, and find a bench in the park. I sit there alone, crying. And I stay there. Alone, unloved, and unattractive. Forever.

This chilling event never happened to Valerie. But anytime she thought about her husband, this worry would start playing in her head. She would try to snuff it out by phoning her husband (always under the pretense of "seeing how your day is going"), pouring herself a drink, checking the credit card bills for unusual expenses, or doing other things to try to assure herself that it wasn't happening. But the more she tried to get rid of this worry, the more it would come back.

Valerie understood that these thoughts were simply a product of her own mind, so she wrote this worry script and read it to herself twice a day, every day, for a week. The first time she read it, she was an emotional wreck. Her fear rating hit 100 and she couldn't even get herself to finish it. Knowing the importance of doing her exposure repeatedly, though, she pulled the script out again later that day. This time it sent her fear rating up to 90, but she was able to read it all the way through.

The next day, the script was still very hard to face (fear rating up to 75), but she started to notice something. She realized that she had never allowed her mind to go all the way through the worry to the point where she ends up alone forever. She always tried to shut it down by calling her husband to check on him. She thought to herself how absurd it was to think that, even if this happened, she would be alone and unloved forever. The second reading of the script that day caused only moderate discomfort (fear rating: 50), and she started to discover other problems with her expectations. Most important, she realized that the "other woman" in her worries was always an incredibly beautiful woman, like a movie star. Was this the standard she was using to decide that she was unattractive?

Over the next several days, Valerie kept reading the script two or three times per day, including the times when she started to feel herself begin to worry about Carl. Each time, the story lost some of its power. She remarked that it was like "watching the same scene from a bad soap opera over and over again." And as she kept reading it, she kept recognizing that it was just a story, not reality. Just because she has that thought doesn't mean that Carl finds her unattractive. Nor does it mean that she *is* unattractive. And it doesn't mean that she's going to be alone and unloved forever. It's just a thought.

After a couple of weeks, Valerie was astonished to discover that the script caused barely any anxiety when she read it. She also found that she was better able to let the thought come and go when she started to worry. As she stopped fighting it, it stopped popping back into her mind. And as she became less bothered by the thought, she was able to stop calling her husband all the time to check up on him.

Bill: Flashbacks of Terror

Bill experienced difficulties with his thoughts in a different way. He had served in the army in combat overseas and had had some terrible experiences, including seeing one of his closest friends get killed right beside him. He had carried that memory with him ever since but never talked to anyone about it. It was simply too hard even to think about. He tried to bury it away in the deepest corners of his mind. For a while he drank a lot and smoked marijuana almost daily to numb the pain.

But Bill couldn't bury the memory. Every time he heard a car backfire, it sounded to him like the bomb that had killed his buddy. Every time he heard a helicopter, it took him back to that horrible day. He even had flashbacks when he saw people dressed in camouflage colors because it reminded him of the war.

When Bill finally got into treatment for PTSD, he knew he had to face his demons. Very reluctantly, he began to allow himself to remember what had happened. Bill felt comfortable using technology and wanted to record his story on his smartphone, but he also jotted down some notes on a piece of paper so that he wouldn't accidentally skip some important details. His trauma story is very affecting and detailed, so be prepared. Here's a small excerpt transcribed from his audio recording (the entire recording was about 15 minutes long when finished):

It is 14:00 hours. Mike and I are on recon, scouting out a possible enemy convoy. Even though we're in the hills, the [expletive] sun is pounding down on us. We're hot, soaked in sweat, and smelling like [expletive]. With all this equipment, guns, and ammunition I am able to reach down and I pull out my binoculars and look up ahead. It's them. A small unit. They are stopped on the side of the road, but I can't see why. There's probably 10 of them, all heavily armed, standing beside two transports.

I signal to Mike to pull back so we can report in to the sergeant. But then my walkie-talkie squelches. Oh [expletive], I think they heard us. We both drop to the ground motionless, poised to protect ourselves. My heart is pounding and I'm trying to hold my breath so they won't hear me. Seconds feel like hours, just waiting for something to happen. Then all hell breaks loose. The dirt around us is torn apart by crackling bullets. Sand and dirt from the bullets hitting ground fly all around. We're going to die. A thousand miles from home. Then it goes quiet. Should we run? Stay? What do we do?

Mike and I stay down. There's too much mess around to see if they bugged out or if they are still there. I look over at Mike to see if he can see anything. He is now 10 feet away from me behind a rock. He's trying to peek over the rock to survey the enemy.

And then he explodes. The [expletive] bastards threw a grenade. The flash is blinding, and the heat sears my skin. I almost pass out from the shock, but I realize I'm covered in blood. It isn't mine. Mike's blood is in my eyes, nose, and mouth. His arm is laying beside me. That's all that remains of Mike. I turn and run. Faster than I have ever run. I don't know where I am going, but I just have to get out of there. Anywhere else but there. I can't tell how long I am running, but I eventually collapse under my own exhaustion in a ravine. I am too tired to move, so I just wait. Covered in Mike's blood. The blood of my best friend. Who I killed because of my radio. Whose body I left out there to rot in this [expletive] wasteland. And now I wait alone, secretly hoping that they will kill me too.

As painful as it was for him, Bill came a long way in his treatment after listening to his script over and over. He was finally able to face his memories of that day. They were still horrible memories, but he learned to accept what had happened and allow it to be part of his past. The nightmares eventually began to subside. He began talking to other veterans about their experiences and found great relief in finally being relieved of this huge weight.

He was even able to start doing exposures to other things that triggered his memories: he'd spend time near a local heliport, watch movies that showed combat, and eventually even went to a memorial for his friend and other fallen soldiers. He knew that he would always be affected by his time in combat, but felt that he was finally able to put Mike to rest.

Rewriting Your Story

A new modification to reliving your memories that is getting attention from psychologists is called "Imagery Rescripting," and it has been showing considerable promise in treatment research. It starts just like you did in the section above—recalling the traumatic memory. But instead of repeatedly listening to or reading the story only, Imagery Rescripting involves three steps:

1. Relive the memory as you did with the exposure.
2. Relive the memory, but as if "current you" is watching "younger you" during the event.
3. Relive the memory as "younger you" but with "older you" there to help you understand what is happening.

The idea is that many traumatic memories are difficult because the individual often feels responsible for some aspect of the event or has misinterpreted some aspect of the event that has stuck in his or her memory. For Bill, the memory of having his buddy Mike die was difficult on its own, but part of the reason the memories were so difficult for Bill was that they also carried a feeling of shame. Bill felt like he had killed Mike because his walkie-talkie made a noise that gave away their position to the enemy.

So, part of Bill's treatment involved Imagery Rescripting. In the first step—with the help of his audio recording—he re-created the memory of that day in his head. He was able to describe the feelings of terror in the moment, but also the feelings of guilt and shame. In the second step, Bill relistened to his recording and relived the story, but imagining his current self safely to the side of the scene watching his younger self. He talked through what "current Bill" could see and understand that "younger Bill" didn't. He saw that there was not enough time between when they saw the convoy and when his walkie-talkie made the loud noise for his younger self to have reached down and turned the walkie-talkie off. They were too busy trying to get hidden so they wouldn't be seen. Plus, "current Bill" was able to recall that those walkie-talkies were notoriously buggy, especially after troops had been crawling around in the heat and dirt.

During the third step, Bill re-created the story once again. This time he was again "younger Bill" but had "current Bill" helping him understand what had happened. In this story, "current Bill" sat with "younger Bill" in the ravine where he had collapsed after running away. "Current Bill" talked to "younger Bill" and explained that the noise from the walkie-talkie wasn't his fault. The same thing could have happened to Mike's walkie-talkie—or the enemy soldiers' walkie-talkies. "Younger Bill" hadn't done anything wrong, and he wouldn't have had time to do anything differently anyway. Bill hadn't killed Mike; wartime enemies did. Finally, "current Bill" reminded "younger Bill" that Mike would have wanted him to get out of there alive rather than getting killed trying to drag his corpse through the desert.

This process was very emotionally draining for Bill at first, but he found it very helpful. Nobody had helped "younger Bill" understand any of these things, so when "younger Bill" showed up in his nightmares he still carried all of the guilt of feeling like he had caused Mike to get killed and shame about having left Mike's body in the desert. But now, both "younger Bill" and "older Bill" were able to see the events in a different light, and they could together put to bed the feelings of guilt and shame that had followed them for years.

Creating Forced-Thought Exposures

While some people have memories or worry stories that repeatedly play out in their heads, others just have images or impulses that jump into consciousness. They may not have a story to write out, but rather just a picture or an urge. They can use what we call "forced-thought exposures."

As the name implies, with this technique you force yourself to have the very thoughts you've been trying not to have. By now you have learned that this kind of counterintuitive act can be amazingly successful because of the way our brains work:

1. If we try to ignore or avoid thoughts, our brain assumes they must be very important thoughts, so it keeps reminding us of them.

2. If, on the other hand, we think about thoughts over and over, our brains become bored with them, just as you become bored if you watch the same episode of a TV show over and over.

You're not trying to turn the nasty thought into a good thought, or an urge to do something terrible into an acceptable thing to do, or a horrific image into a pleasant image. The goal of forced-thought exposures is to allow the thought simply to be a thought—a ho-hum, run-of-the-mill thought like any other that might drift through your head without causing you to feel extreme anxiety.

When creating your forced-thought Exposure Plan, there are several questions to think about:

- "Do I have many different images or urges that I need to confront or just one?"
- "Are there any situations in which I have that thought and then feel either better or worse?"
- "If my scary thoughts are about other people, are the thoughts about any particular person more upsetting than my thoughts about others?"
- "Are there any other factors that might make some exposures easier or harder than others?"

As with all exposures, one of the most important parts is to break it down into manageable chunks and start with the easier parts first. That's what Wendy did.

Wendy and the Image of Her Brother

Wendy keeps seeing horrific images of her brother, Steve, as a dead, mutilated body lying on the ground—despite the fact that Steve is very much alive and well. As much as she hates these images, she also fears that they imply she secretly wants her brother dead or even wants to kill him. In fact, she moved out of her family's home and into an apartment because she was scared that she might lose control and harm Steve. She thinks she's an awful person for having these thoughts, and she tries to force the images out of her mind by thinking of other things. That never worked, so she drew up an Exposure Plan; see Sample Completed Form 8.3 (Wendy).

To start her Exposure Plan, Wendy decided that she would intentionally picture her brother's body while she was in her apartment and her brother was at home with their parents. That way, she felt that (1) she couldn't accidentally lose control and hurt him and (2) her parents would be around in case he somehow did get hurt.

SAMPLE COMPLETED FORM 8.3 (Wendy)

Exposure Plan in Order of Difficulty

Rank order	Fear trigger: Situation, object, thought, or sensations	Fear rating (0–100)
1	Picturing the image when I'm with my brother and something is nearby that could be used as a weapon (for example, a kitchen knife)	100
2	Picturing the image when I'm alone with my brother (no weapon)	95
3	Picturing the image when I'm with my brother, but our parents are also around	90
4	Picturing the image at a time when I know my brother isn't at home	85
5	Picturing the image at a time when my brother is at home alone	70
6	Picturing the image at a time when my brother is at home and with my parents	60

She decided that she would picture the image for 20 minutes twice a day. She also remembered about safety behaviors (Chapter 8) and decided that she would not call Steve afterward to see if he was okay. After the first 20-minute exposure, Wendy's fear rating was around 90 and she really wanted to call to check on her brother. Fortunately, she resisted checking, and after about 45 minutes her anxiety had come back down to normal.

The second time she did the exposure that day the image didn't cause her as much trouble. Her fear rating went up to only 60, and it came back down to normal within 20 minutes. She did experience some anxiety before going to sleep because she really wanted to call Steve to hear his voice. But she knew she shouldn't. Wendy practiced that exposure twice a day all week, and by the end of the week the image didn't bother her much because she knew that her brother was safe at home with their parents.

Wendy continued to practice the items on her Exposure Plan, gradually working her way up to the more difficult ones. She pictured the image when she knew her brother was home alone for a week and then pictured it when she knew he was outside. These exposures were hard to do at first, but by the end of the week her fear ratings had always gone back down. Wendy still felt scared about being with her brother while experiencing the thought, worried that she might hurt him. But she no longer feared that just having the thought might somehow cause him to be harmed. To her surprise, she also realized that, other than the times when she was doing her exposure practices, the picture wasn't popping into her mind very often anymore!

Because Wendy and Steve were very close, she told him about these thoughts. Her brother didn't seem upset by them and, after teasing her a little, gladly agreed to help her out with the remaining exposures. They made a plan: Wendy would come over in the evening on days when their parents would be home and force herself to imagine the picture while in the room with Steve. Although this exposure upset Wendy the first time, with her fear rating going up to 100, the second time was much easier.

It became clear to her that there was no way she would lose control and turn into the "fratricidal maniac" she feared. Realizing this, Wendy and Steve conducted a series of exposures in which Wendy brought on the feared image when they were alone together with several kitchen knives in the room. None of the remaining exposures set off Wendy's anxiety.

Now, a year later, Wendy almost never has that image pop into her head. And the rare times when she does think about it, the picture doesn't upset her because she knows it's just a "stupid thought." She sometimes even plays with the mental picture. She imagines the corpse getting up and dancing the cha-cha-cha as a way of reminding herself that it is a silly, meaningless image.

Exposure to Uncertainty

If you are fearful of or anxious about uncertainty in general, the most effective approach is to focus on exposing yourself to uncertainty. This doesn't mean exposure to every situation or possibility that might come into your mind—nobody has time for that!—but rather to do exposures to uncertainty in general to build up your tolerance for it. This might involve picking a new restaurant to try without looking up any reviews and showing up without a reservation, making a quick decision about a minor matter without researching the "best" solution, or taking a new route home from work even though you don't know what the traffic will be like. The goal isn't to find a new route or to get better at picking restaurants; it's to become more tolerant of feelings of uncertainty and learning that catastrophic things won't happen if you don't pick the right solution.

In addition, when life throws you opportunities to build your tolerance for uncertainty, these are great exposures. If you have a paper due for a class, this is an opportunity to do an exposure by writing it, proofreading it only once, and handing it in. If you receive a letter from the tax office, do an exposure by waiting 3 days to open it and sitting with the uncertainty of what the letter might say.

As with all exposures, it is very important that you not use your safety behaviors to cope. This might mean not double-checking or triple-checking your work for mistakes. Or asking someone for reassurance. Or procrastinating on making decisions. Take the story of James, for example.

James: The Quest for Certainty

James was a middle-aged professional who had worked in corporate finance for many years. Others often described him as a perfectionist, but he saw himself more as being afraid of making mistakes and taking chances. In some ways this had helped him professionally—he very rarely made mistakes in his financial reports, but he always seemed to work twice as long as everyone else in the office. More often than not, James took work home with him and spent his evenings reviewing his spreadsheets, recomputing expenses and assets, and scrutinizing his reports for errors. And while he was usually very accurate, many of his reports were late because of his checking. James had been passed over for promotion several times because of this. One time when he was offered a minor promotion, his managers withdrew the offer after he had not responded within 2 weeks. James had procrastinated over making a decision about it because he was unsure about what the extra duties might be and whether he would be able to handle them.

Outside of work—or at least during the little time that James wasn't working—he really wanted to develop a romantic relationship. His marriage had ended several years ago, partly because of the amount of time he spent working. He had downloaded one of those "swipe left/right" dating apps on his phone but would stay up late in bed scrutinizing every profile for hours. He would worry about whether the information each woman had written about herself might mean that they wouldn't be a good match or whether what she had written was inaccurate, but then would worry that if he swiped left (saying he wasn't interested) that he might miss out on meeting the love of his life. Needless to say, he wasn't very successful in getting matches because of his fear of uncertainty.

Frustrated by his problems at work and in his love life, James eventually made the decision to face his fear of uncertainty head-on. That decision actually took quite a long time, because James kept trying to gather more and more information on which treatment approach was best. When he did make the decision to try exposure to uncertainty, he realized that making the decision was actually his first exposure! As James was still skeptical about facing uncertainty in his financial work, he decided to start his exposures on the dating scene. The dating app James was using didn't allow you to go back and change your "interested" or "not interested" swipes, so he saw this as an opportunity to make quick decisions that were final. He made a deal with himself that he would make a decision about each woman's profile within 5 minutes and then swipe one way or the other. Initially, his anxiety would go up to 80 as his timer closed in on 5 minutes and he would simply swipe "not interested" on almost every one, but he found that he wouldn't perseverate on whether he had missed out on a perfect date for very long. So he started allowing himself to swipe "interested" more and more and also found that his ability to tolerate the uncertainty about whether they would "like" him back increased. In fact, several women did match with him! He chatted for a couple of weeks with a woman he liked, and they decided to meet in person. James took this opportunity to increase his exposure to uncertainty and picked a small café for their first meeting even though he had never been there before.

Following up on his success in tolerating uncertainty regarding his love life, James felt it was time to start trying to apply these exposures to uncertainty around his work. Unfortunately, this was much harder for him because he worried that if his reports were not perfect, he might get fired. And that would open up a world of uncertainty! So he decided to reduce his checking and reviewing gradually. Instead of reviewing his spreadsheets and reports for 3 or 4 hours every evening, he would start by limiting this to just 2 hours at first. He decided that if he hadn't found any errors after 2 hours, there probably weren't any errors. This was quite difficult for James during the first week, and his anxiety often went up to 70. But to his surprise, his managers didn't find any errors on his reports and calculations. James's colleague did catch one slight mistake—he had forgotten to add one small expense—but this was easily corrected. James was embarrassed about making the mistake but took heart that a simple and easily fixable error was the only consequence of reducing his checking.

At this point, James has reduced his at-home checking to just 1 hour, which gets his anxiety up to a 50 at most. He is feeling quite excited about how well he has reduced his fear of uncertainty, particularly because he now has more free time in the evenings to spend with that lovely woman he met on the dating app!

Troubleshooting

Exposures to thoughts, memories, images, urges, and uncertainty can be a wonderfully effective tool in your attempts to overcome your anxiety, but they do present a challenge. The nature of the exercise means that you must confront some very distressing thoughts, and breaking the entrenched habit of avoiding frightening thoughts is no easy task. Changing your way of thinking is one big stride toward success; remember that a frightening thought doesn't mean something bad is going to happen. Nor does a traumatic memory mean that you're about to experience a trauma again. And frightening thoughts or urges don't mean that you are a bad person! A thought is just a thought.

A thought is just a thought.

Some people even use a phrase like that as a kind of mantra in their quest to free themselves of their anxious thoughts, reminding themselves again and again: *A thought is just a thought*. It helps them cope with the distress they feel when doing forced-thought exposures or exposure to worry/trauma scripts.

Finally, if you find yourself having trouble doing these exposures, don't get discouraged. Scale back and start with a thought or memory that's a little easier to manage, then keep moving forward bit by bit. Maybe you can start with just part of the memory and add more pieces later. Perhaps you can start with less detail and then add in more later. You'll be surprised at how much easier it gets. As a friend once said, "Doing exposures repeatedly is therapy; doing exposure once is torture." Each time you practice the exposure, it will cause you less distress and give you more benefit. Trust us—the improvements you make will be well worth your efforts.

11

confronting frightening feelings and sensations

Almost everyone experiences intense physical symptoms when frightened. This chapter is for that smaller group of people who are frightened by the sensations themselves. You should read this chapter closely if your Exposure Plan included facing bodily sensations that cause you anxiety. This could involve a fear of any number of feelings or sensations, including:

- ☑ Racing or pounding heart
- ☑ Shortness of breath
- ☑ Blushing
- ☑ Headache or other pains
- ☑ Numbness or tingling sensations
- ☑ Nausea or upset stomach

- ☑ Dizziness or lightheadedness
- ☑ Feeling "shaky" or trembling
- ☑ Hot flashes or chills
- ☑ Feeling weak-kneed
- ☑ Sweating
- ☑ Choking feelings

Different people may fear the same feelings for completely different reasons. Take feelings of sweatiness, for example. An individual with panic disorder might fear sweating as a sign of impending panic attack. Another person with health anxiety might fear it because it's a symptom of malaria. Someone with social fears might fear it because other people might see it as a sign that she is nervous. People with obsessive–compulsive contamination concerns might fear sweating because it makes them feel slimy and gross. No matter the cause, if such feelings activate your anxiety, avoiding them is not the answer.

The Effects of Avoiding Frightening Sensations

You may be asking yourself, "If I don't like that sensation and I can avoid it, why shouldn't I?" This is one of the most common concerns raised by people who have fears related to bodily sensations. If having a racing heart scares you and makes you think you're having a heart attack, why should you do anything that makes your heart race? Well, there are three important reasons for *not* avoiding the sensations you fear.

> *If I don't like that sensation and I can avoid it, why shouldn't I?*

1. The sensations you fear represent normal bodily functions. Our bodies are designed to perform certain tasks and to experience certain feelings that keep us functioning properly every day. Our hearts beat faster when our bodies need blood to circulate more quickly (for example, during exercise, when feeling frightened, or for a number of other reasons). We sweat when our bodies detect that we're starting to overheat. We tremble if we're frightened because our bodies release adrenaline. These are all feelings that are very difficult to control because they are expressions of normal physical functions. These sensations happen regardless of how hard we try *not* to feel them.

2. Avoiding sensations increases your awareness of them over time. By trying to avoid sensations, we actually make it more likely that we'll feel them at a later time. This process is a lot like what happened in the "Spotty the Polar Bear" exercise in Chapter 10. When we try to avoid something because it scares us, our brains are designed to lock on to an image of that very thing.

And this makes sense. If you were scared because you thought a cougar was prowling around your neighborhood, your brain would shift into "cougar-detection mode." Every time you heard a rustle in the bushes, your brain would scan and ask, "Is that a cougar?" If you saw something moving out of the corner of your eye, your brain would scan and ask, "Is that a cougar?" Normally this reaction is a good thing. You would be extra likely to spot the cougar if it were actually there. And that might give you the extra warning you need to get away from it safely.

But what about sensations that our bodies produce when they're not on high alert? Most of the time we don't notice these run-of-the-mill sensations. If you're sitting down right now, take a moment to notice the feelings of your rear on the chair. Feel your back press against the back of the seat. Before you started thinking about those feelings, you probably didn't even notice them. But does that mean those feelings weren't there before? No, you just weren't paying attention to them.

The fact is that our bodies produce hundreds of different sensations every second. There's the little gurgle in your stomach as you digest food, the beating of your heart, the feeling of air entering and leaving your lungs, the pressure of your shoes on your feet, an itch on your cheek, the taste of saliva in your mouth. We rarely notice such sensations, but if they were to scare us, we would scan for them constantly. And because those sensations are normally there, we'd notice them. And that would scare us.

3. Efforts to avoid sensations can trigger them instead. The third, and possibly most important, reason that trying to avoid sensations doesn't work is that by avoiding those sensations you often conjure them up! Consider Teresa's story.

Teresa and her husband are in their early 40s. Both are healthy eaters with active lifestyles. Unexpectedly, Teresa's husband had a mild heart attack and, although he survived and is doing fine now, the experience terrified Teresa. "If he could have a heart attack despite his healthy lifestyle, I guess I could too," she thought. Since her husband's heart attack, Teresa has been paying close attention to her body for signs.

One evening while watching TV, she thought she noticed her heart beating faster. "Oh my God, is this a heart attack?" she immediately thought. Obviously this possibility scared Teresa. Remember back to the beginning of this book where you read about how your body shifts into "fight-or-flight" mode when you're frightened? One of the first things your body does when in fight-or-flight mode is to release adrenaline to make your heart beat faster.

For Teresa, a racing heart leads to the thought that she is dying. This thought scares her even more, which increases the intensity of her fight-or-flight response. This might trigger an even faster heartbeat, as well as other sensations, such as shortness of breath or tingling in her fingers and toes. What do you predict Teresa would think if she noticed those sensations? Would those thoughts make her more scared? And if she did get more scared, what would happen to her fight-or-flight feelings?

Right—they'd get even worse! The fact that Teresa is so afraid of her heart beating rapidly is precisely what caused her heart to start beating rapidly in the first place. This loop in which fear causes symptoms and symptoms strengthen fears can produce all kinds of perfectly natural sensations that can become linked to fears. Shortness of breath can set off people with claustrophobia. Shakiness can upset people who fear that others will see them looking nervous. Those so-called butterflies in your stomach can frighten people who fear they might throw up or lose control of their bowels. Feelings of lightheadedness can bother people who are afraid of passing out.

> **Repeat 5 times fast:**
>
> **Fears of feelings can cause the feelings that fuel the fears!**

As a final point, what do you think would have happened to Teresa if her heart had started to beat a little bit faster a month *before* her husband's heart attack? Would she even have noticed it? Possibly not. And even if she had, it probably wouldn't have upset her. At that point, she wasn't even considering the possibility of a heart attack. She might have thought her racing heart was prompted by a cup of coffee, walking around quickly, or being excited about something—and none of these thoughts would have scared her. Because she isn't scared of these thoughts, she wouldn't have experienced a fight-or-flight response, and her heart wouldn't have sped up even more.

So, at the risk of giving you an impossible tongue twister, the point is that *fears of feelings can cause the feelings that fuel the fears*.

Exposing Yourself to Frightening Feelings and Sensations

The methods for exposure to objects and situations, and even to thoughts or memories, may seem more obvious than do the methods for exposure to sensations in your body. After all, if you fear heights, you should go to a high place. If you fear memories of a car accident, think about the car accident. But if you fear feeling short of breath, how do you make yourself feel that way?

It's easier than you might think. Psychologists and other mental health professionals have developed a number of simple activities that can safely induce a variety of unusual sensations.

These activities are called *interoceptive exercises*. "Interoception" refers to the process of feeling sensations inside your body, such as your heart beating or your muscles tightening. Interoceptive exercises are designed to create those different internal feelings.

The steps involved in exposures to bodily sensations are exactly the same as the exposure exercises you learned in Chapter 8. After you decide, based on your Exposure Plan, that you're going to do exposures to bodily sensations, you will:

1. Plan the details of how you will bring on the sensation
2. Practice challenging the thoughts you're likely to experience during the exposure
3. Set specific measurable goals based on actions, not feelings
4. Start the exposure practice
5. Stay in the exposure until your anxiety decreases
6. Avoid using any safety behaviors or safety thoughts
7. Finish the exposure practice
8. Review your goals and assess whether any of your anxious thoughts or expectations came true
9. Reward yourself for facing your fears

The box below through page 193 describes some common interoceptive exercises and the sensations most frequently reported during each one.

Before you start, you should know that for most people these exercises are perfectly safe, though they may trigger uncomfortable feelings. Which is exactly the point. But for some people, there may be medical reasons why these exercises might not be advisable. Several years ago, one of our colleagues, Dr. Steven Taylor, consulted a prominent physician and developed a list of

Common Interoceptive Exercises

Interoceptive exercise	How it works	Strongest sensations usually triggered
Breathe through a straw or breathe while pursing your lips	Breathe through a small straw (a small drinking straw or a stir straw for coffee) for 2 minutes. Hold your nose so that you don't "cheat." This exercise produces a sensation that you are not getting enough air into your lungs.	Breathlessness/smothering sensations Pounding/racing heart Choking
Hold your head between your knees, then lift your head up quickly	While sitting, bend forward and put your head between your legs. If possible, keep your head lower than your rear. Stay like this for 30 seconds, then sit up quickly.	Dizziness or faint feelings Breathlessness/smothering sensations

Interoceptive exercise	How it works	Strongest sensations usually triggered
Hold your head between your knees, then lift your head up quickly *(continued)*	This exercise works by pushing extra blood into your head. When you sit up, your blood pours back into the rest of your body giving a temporary feeling called a "head rush."	Numbness/tingling in face or extremities
Hold your breath	Hold your breath for 30 seconds. This exercise works by setting off alarms in your body that are designed to detect changes in the amount of oxygen and carbon dioxide in your system.	Breathlessness/smothering sensations Pounding/racing heart Dizziness or fainting feelings
Hyperventilate	Breathe very quickly and very deeply for 1 minute. Pretend you are trying to blow up a balloon very quickly. This exercise works by setting off alarms in your body that are designed to detect changes in the amount of oxygen and carbon dioxide in your system.	Breathlessness/smothering sensations Dizziness or fainting feelings Pounding/racing heart Numbness/tingling in face or extremities
Run in place	Run in place for 1 minute, as if you're jogging. If you have home exercise stair-step blocks, you could also stair-step for 1 minute. As does any form of aerobic exercise, this works by increasing your heart and breathing rates.	Pounding/racing heart Breathlessness/smothering sensations Chest pain/tightness
Sit facing a heater	Sit 2 feet in front of a small space heater for 2 minutes. This works simply by overheating the body. The hot air also makes it feel more difficult to breathe.	Breathlessness/smothering sensations Sweating Hot flushes/chills
Spin in a chair	Sitting in a swivel chair, spin around for 1 minute. This exercise works by temporarily confusing your vestibular apparatus, a part of your inner ear that helps control balance.	Dizziness or fainting feelings Pounding/racing heart Breathlessness/smothering sensations Nausea

Interoceptive exercise	How it works	Strongest sensations usually triggered
Stare at a light and then read	Stare at a ceiling light for 1 minute. Then immediately try to read a book or magazine. Staring at the light causes your pupils to constrict to adapt to the extra light. It also saturates some of the receptors on the retina with light.	Blurred vision Dizziness or fainting feelings Feeling unreal or in a dream
Stare at a mirror	Stare directly into your own eyes in a mirror for 2 minutes. Staring at the same spot for a long time can create odd perceptual experiences and a "tunnel vision" effect.	Feeling unreal or as if in a dream Dizziness or fainting feelings
Stare at a rotating spiral	Using the Internet, find a video of a rotating spiral, for example, *www.youtube.com/watch?v=XYOSK9stBAU* Stare at the center of the spiral as intently as you can for 3 minutes. Staring at the center spot for a long time can create odd perceptual experiences and a "tunnel vision" effect.	Feeling unreal or in a dream Dizziness or fainting feelings
Tense your muscles	Tense up every muscle in your body—your face, shoulders, arms, trunk, legs, and feet—as tightly as you can for 1 minute. Holding muscles tense will cause them to shake while the muscles strain to maintain the contractions. Tensing the muscles through your torso also makes it feel more difficult to breathe.	Trembling/shaking Breathlessness/smothering sensations Pounding/racing heart
Use a tongue depressor	Using a Popsicle stick or a wooden tongue depressor like your doctor uses, press down on the back of your tongue for 30 seconds. This exercise works by stimulating nerves in the back of your throat that are part of your gag reflex.	Gagging or choking Breathlessness/smothering sensations Nausea/abdominal distress

potential medical reasons why certain interoceptive exercises should be avoided. The box below outlines some of these contraindications. If you're concerned about hurting yourself when doing any of these exercises, review this list with your physician to be sure they're safe for you. If you have any medical problems or physical limitations (for example, high or low blood pressure, asthma, a cold or chest infection, heart disease, migraines, seizure disorders, and so on), talk to your doctor before practicing these exercises.

Try each of these exercises to see which ones might set off your anxiety. Previous research has found that the ones that most consistently bring on feelings of anxiety and fear include breathing through a straw, spinning in a chair, and hyperventilating. Each of these exercises is effective for at least some people, so it's worth trying as many as you can at least once. Use Form 11.1 to rate each exercise in terms of how much fear or distress it produced for you, from

Contraindications for Certain Interoceptive Exercises

Interoceptive Exercise	Potential Contraindications
■ Breathe through a straw or breathe while pursing your lips	☑ Chronic obstructive pulmonary disease
■ Hold your head between your knees, then lift your head up quickly	☑ Postural hypotension, lower back pain, history of falling due to dizziness or balance disorder
■ Hold your breath	☑ Chronic obstructive pulmonary disease
■ Hyperventilate	☑ Chronic obstructive pulmonary disease, severe asthma, cardiac conditions, epilepsy, renal disease, pregnancy
■ Run in place	☑ Cardiac conditions, severe asthma, lower back pain, pregnancy
■ Sit facing a heater	☑ No apparent contraindications
■ Spin in a chair	☑ Pregnancy, history of falling due to dizziness or balance disorder
■ Stare at a light and then read	☑ Light sensitivity (photophobia)
■ Stare at a mirror	☑ No apparent contraindications
■ Stare at a rotating spiral	☑ No apparent contraindications
■ Tense your muscles	☑ Pain disorders; if pain is localized, patients could tense all but the affected region
■ Use a tongue depressor	☑ Prominent gag reflex (stimulation of which will induce vomiting)

FORM 11.1

Rating the Exercises

Interoceptive Exposure Plan		
Interoceptive exercise	**Fear rating (0–100)**	**Rank order (1–12)**
Breathe through a straw or while pursing your lips		
Hold head between knees then lift head quickly		
Hold breath		
Hyperventilate		
Run in place		
Sit facing heater		
Spin in a chair		
Stare at light and then read		
Stare at a mirror		
Stare at a rotating spiral, for example, *www.youtube.com/watch?v=XYOSK9stBAU*		
Tense muscles		
Use a tongue depressor		

0 (no effect) to 100 (causing an extreme amount of fear). Once you have them all rated, go back and rank them from least difficult to most difficult (12 to 1).

Look back over Form 11.1 and cross out any exercises that didn't cause your anxiety to go over 30. Then find the lowest-ranked exercise that remains and make it the first one you practice regularly. Each time, after you've finished the exercise, write down how anxious it made you feel, using the same 0 (none) to 100 (extreme fear) scale. Keep practicing your chosen exercise until it doesn't cause your anxiety to rise over 30. Then you should move up to the next-highest-ranked exercise and repeat the process.

If you can, practice each exercise twice a day, every day. At the very least, practice it once a day. Naturally, improvements will be quicker with more frequent practice. You can also create your own exercises to bring on the feelings you fear. If you're frightened of your legs feeling shaky and "rubbery" when you are anxious, for example, try completing a series of squats until your legs feel weak and rubbery. It's easy to find instructions online if you need them.

Combining Interoceptive and Situational Exposures

For some people, like Deborah, the interoceptive exercises alone are not enough to trigger fear. Deborah had panic attacks for many years, and she particularly feared feeling breathless. Deborah had learned, however, that her panicky feelings would subside quickly either if she was alone or if she could leave the situation to get some time by herself. She felt particularly optimistic about the hyperventilation, straw-breathing, and breath-holding exercises since they were supposed to trigger feelings such as shortness of breath and smothering sensations.

Unfortunately, Deborah found that doing the exercises at home alone wasn't making her anxious. She recognized that she needed to practice these exercises in places where she wasn't alone, especially places from which she couldn't easily escape if she started to feel anxious. So she bought some coffee stir straws and decided to practice straw breathing while in the mall. She started out at less busy times and eventually worked up to straw breathing for 2 minutes during the busy weekend shopping hours. She later practiced holding her breath since this was an exercise she could do in public without anyone noticing. She also attended a professional basketball game and climbed the stairs to her seat very rapidly—an inconspicuous alternative to running in place.

Here are some other examples of how you might combine interoceptive exercises with situational exposure practices for various types of fears:

- Spin around in a chair for a minute to get dizzy and then look out the window of a high building (fear of being dizzy in high places)

- Wear a heavy sweater during a presentation (fear of sweating while speaking in public)

- Hyperventilate in a small closet (fear of feeling lightheaded in enclosed places)

- Drink hot soup while in the presence of a group of other people (fear of feeling hot and flushed in social situations)

- Purposely make your hands shake while filling out a check or lottery ticket at a store (fear of having shaky hands in public)

- Wear a scarf or tie while flying in an airplane (fear of tightness in the throat while flying)

Troubleshooting

Like all exposure exercises, exposure to frightening feelings and sensations can be difficult and distressing at first—they *have* to be in order to work. But bear with them, because with time they will get easier and easier. Before long you won't even react to the feelings or sensations. Encourage yourself by imagining the time when they will be no more anxiety provoking than any other sensation your body produces. Make a commitment to your goal and you'll achieve it.

ADDITIONAL STRATEGIES

Welcome to Part III, the final section of the book. We hope that by this point you have overcome some or all of the difficulties you were experiencing with anxiety. If you haven't quite made the progress you had hoped for in Part II, feel free to go back and continue working on the thought-challenging skills (Chapters 5, 6, and 7) and the exposure exercises (Chapters 8, 9, 10, and 11). Part III will still be here when you are ready.

In Part III, we present additional skills that some people find helpful in dealing with stress and residual anxiety. We don't consider them part of the core program, but they can be useful additional strategies. In Chapter 12, you will learn some relaxation skills to help you deal with stress, general worries, and mild anxiety. You will learn two types of relaxation: *progressive muscle relaxation* and *breathing retraining*. We encourage you to try both of these for about a week each to see if you find either or both helpful. We have made available to you audio recordings of the progressive muscle relaxation exercises. Feel free to download these to your mobile device or music player (see the box at the end of the Contents for information on where to access these files, and see page 246 for a list of audio tracks).

Chapter 13 introduces you to *mindfulness* strategies. These exercises, which are currently very popular, may be helpful for dealing with stress and residual anxiety after you complete the program. We recommend you also read this chapter and practice the strategies for about a week. If you find them helpful, you can continue practicing them. In Chapter 13 we also recommend books on mindfulness-related strategies in case you want to explore this topic in more detail.

Finally, in the Conclusion you will take a look back at all of the gains you have made and learn about strategies to maintain these improvements over the long run. You will also develop strategies for dealing with occasional lapses and obtain information on how to address the possibility of your anxiety returning. We hope that it won't—and it usually doesn't—but it is important to be prepared. Finally, at the end of the book we have included a comprehensive list of resources, including ways to find a therapist or more information on anxiety, digital and online tools for working on your anxiety, and other books that we recommend.

12

learning to relax

If your anxiety stems from life stresses, such as work difficulties or relationship problems, you may benefit from the techniques described in this chapter. Relaxation-based strategies are often used along with the other techniques described in this book, including thought challenging (Chapters 5–7) and exposure (Chapters 8–11). They're particularly helpful for generalized anxiety disorder (GAD) and managing day-to-day stress. If, after having practiced thought challenging and exposure you still feel some degree of general anxiety or stress, see if these exercises can reduce your tension even more.

Relaxation techniques ideally should not be used before or during exposures for the same reason we don't want you to use avoidance strategies; you need to learn that the objects or situations that provoke your anxiety are manageable and not as dangerous as you believed. Using relaxation before or during exposures teaches your brain that the situations or objects are manageable because you used your relaxation skills, not because they aren't as dangerous as you had believed. Learning and using relaxation at other times may help to take the edge off your day-to-day anxiety, worry, and stress.

Do not use relaxation before or during exposures!

In this chapter you'll learn about two types of relaxation-based strategies, progressive muscle relaxation and breathing retraining. (Readers interested in a more detailed discussion of relaxation-based approaches to dealing with anxiety should check out the seventh edition of the *Relaxation and Stress Reduction Workbook* by Martha Davis and colleagues.) In the next chapter, we'll also talk about mindfulness- and acceptance-based strategies for anxiety. (A more detailed review of these strategies can be found in the second edition of *The Mindfulness and Acceptance Workbook for Anxiety* by John Forsyth and Georg Eifert.) These books are listed in the Resources.

Feel free to try both the progressive muscle relaxation and the breathing retraining to see which you prefer for reducing your stress and anxiety. Each has its own advantages, and there is no evidence that doing both will reduce your stress any more than just doing one or the other, so go with whichever is most helpful for you. In our experience, some people prefer breathing retraining because it can be done easily and discreetly, but others have said that they dislike it because it doesn't feel engaging—that their minds tend to wander and negative thoughts can creep in. Progressive muscle relaxation, on the other hand, is a very active process that can keep your mind focused on the activities. But as you may have guessed, it is more involved and generally requires you to go to a quiet room with a comfortable chair. Both seem to work equally well, so feel free to pick whichever tends to work best for you.

Progressive Muscle Relaxation

Progressive muscle relaxation (PMR) is a very popular relaxation technique involving a series of exercises in which you first tense a particular muscle group and then relax it. The alternating phases make you aware of how different your muscles feel when they're tense versus when they're relaxed. People who use PMR report that the exercises help alert them to muscle tension early on, before it becomes intense and more difficult to undo.

The series of exercises takes 15 or 20 minutes initially. At the beginning, PMR involves alternately tensing (for about 10 seconds) and relaxing (for about 20 seconds) 12 muscle groups, one at a time. We call this "long-form" PMR. Once you become better at achieving a relaxed state, you can move to "short-form" PMR, which involves tensing and relaxing several muscle groups at once, for a total of five tension–relaxation cycles. After you practice long-form and short-form PMR for a number of weeks, you will be better at recognizing what it feels like to be tense versus relaxed, and it will be easier to let go of your tension in one simple step lasting just a few seconds. This final step is what we call "full-body" PMR, which involves tensing all of your muscles at once and then relaxing. You can download our audio recordings of the relaxation scripts for all three versions of PMR (see the box at the end of the Contents for information on where to access these files, and see page 246 for a list of audio tracks). They are based on an excellent set of instructions developed by Dr. Debra Hope and narrated by Dr. Timothy Jones and used with their permission.

Here are a few suggestions to keep in mind:

■ Set aside time to practice your relaxation every day. We recommend practicing each script, beginning with the long form, for 2 weeks until you have completed all of the scripts. This will give you plenty of practice time to become very good at achieving a deep state of relaxation.

■ Complete the Progressive Muscle Relaxation Progress Form (Form 12.1) for each relaxation practice. Before each practice, rate your level of anxiety from 0 (no anxiety) to 100 (worst imaginable anxiety). After the practice, record your anxiety or tension level again, using the same scale. Keep a record of these ratings to follow your progress.

■ There are a few steps you can take to increase your level of relaxation, especially in the first few practices. Be sure to practice with your eyes closed while sitting in a comfortable chair (a recliner is ideal). Turn off the telephone, dim the lights, and wear comfortable clothing with a loose collar. If you wear a smartwatch, either take it off or set it to "Do Not Disturb" mode. After a few weeks of practice, you don't have to go to these lengths—after all, the long-term goal is to be able to feel relaxed no matter where you are or what you are doing.

Progressive Muscle Relaxation Progress Form

Mark your ratings on a scale from 0 (no anxiety) to 100 (worst imaginable anxiety).		
Date/time	Anxiety/tension before	Anxiety/tension after

■ Once you become more comfortable conducting the relaxation exercises while listening to the script, try going through the exercises without listening to it. This will require you to memorize the exercises, though you don't have to do them in exactly the same order as in the script. Conducting the exercises without listening to the script will help you to relax on your own, without requiring you to have someone with you or any special equipment to play the instructions.

■ As you move through the exercises, try to stay focused on your muscles, your breathing, and your state of relaxation. If any other thoughts pop into your mind, just let them go. Don't fight your thoughts or feelings. Be aware of them and then let them go.

■ If there are sounds in the room, such as the buzzing of lights or traffic noise in the distance, just let them go as well. Gently bring your attention back to the exercise.

■ Some people may feel increased anxiety or even panicky feelings early in treatment, especially those who feel anxious when focusing on the feelings in their bodies. With practice, the exercises usually become more relaxing and less likely to trigger discomfort.

Were you able to reduce your anxiety? If not, keep trying!

You should practice with the audio file Progressive Muscle Relaxation—Long Form (track 1) every day for 2 weeks to get the most benefit from it (see the box at the end of the Contents for information on where to access this and the other files). Learning to relax is a skill, just like learning to play the piano or learning to swim. Don't expect it to work perfectly the first time. Just keep practicing. Most experts recommend practicing once or twice daily. Soon you'll find that you're developing good control over your feelings of anxiety and tension.

After 2 weeks of practicing the long form of the script, when you find it easier to become relaxed, try the short form of PMR, the Progressive Muscle Relaxation—Short Form audio file, or track 2. Make sure you continue rating your anxiety/tension before and after you practice relaxing. Once you're comfortable completing the exercises while listening to the instruction, try practicing without listening to it.

Keep practicing the short version every day, again for 2 weeks. Then, for a final step, move to the full-body version, or Progressive Muscle Relaxation—Full Body (audio track 3). It's brief and easy to use when you don't have a lot of time. Begin your practices in a relaxing environment (eyes closed, comfortable chair and clothing, quiet room), and gradually progress to practicing in less relaxing environments.

Valerie—Relaxing Her Mind and Body

Valerie, the woman who had constant worries about a range of things—her husband's safety in particular—decided that she wanted to try out PMR. She had mostly overcome her worries and was continuing to practice her exposures but found that she was still tense and stressed fairly often due to her work demands. She downloaded the three audio recordings to her phone and scheduled a half hour at home every morning before work to practice her relaxation. She moved a comfortable lounge chair into her spare bedroom and asked her husband, Carl, not to interrupt her during this time. She also turned her phone to "Do Not Disturb" mode so she wouldn't get distracted by any texts, calls, or e-mails.

Valerie immediately found the voice of the narrator to be extremely soothing, and she really liked the experience of tensing and relaxing her muscles one by one until she felt, in her own words, "like warm butter." After completing the long form of PMR for the first time, she noted how much less stressed she was about going to work, so she also decided that she would practice her relaxation a second time each day in the evening. After about a week of using the long-form recording, she decided to switch to the short form and practiced that twice per day for another week. She continued to practice her exposures as well, but remembered that she shouldn't use relaxation before or during the exposures.

Finally, Valerie tried the full-body version of the audio recordings. She found that she could easily get herself quite relaxed using this, especially when at work. But she realized that she preferred the short-form version, because it let her have about 20 minutes of time to herself. So she kept practicing the short form twice every day, once in the morning and once in the evening, but continued to use the full-body techniques periodically throughout the week when she would feel stress about meetings or deadlines at work.

Breathing Retraining

You may have noticed that when you're under a lot of stress or anxiety your breathing becomes more rapid and shallow. This can sometimes lead to shortness of breath, a normal component of the fight-or-flight response (discussed in Chapter 1). Unlike other changes that occur during the fight-or-flight response (for example, the release of adrenaline, changes in heart rate, changes in liver activity), breathing is under our own control. In fact, breathing is one of the few systems in the body that is both involuntary (it keeps going even if you aren't thinking about it, such as when you are asleep) and voluntary (you can directly control it, such as by blowing or holding your breath). So when the fight-or-flight response instigates sped-up breathing through the *involuntary* system, you can regain control of your breath by using a *voluntary* override.

How Does Breathing Work?

A silly question . . . our lungs suck in air and then blow it back out, right? That's how many people think about their breathing—and it's entirely false. We don't actually have any muscles in our lungs for sucking in air or blowing it back out. Believe it or not, our lungs are essentially glorified grocery bags. Breathing comes from two groups of muscles that don't even touch the lungs. Instead, they expand or shrink our chest "cavity," which is the inside part of our bodies, extending from the shoulders roughly down to the stomach.

These groups of muscles are the *intercostal muscles* and the *diaphragm*. The intercostals are a series of muscles that line the rib cage. The diaphragm is a large muscle that completely separates the upper part of the inside of your body from your abdomen, which houses the stomach, intestines, and so on. The main job of the intercostals is to expand and contract the rib cage. The job of the diaphragm, which is shaped like a dome or an upside-down bowl, is to flatten itself. Why would they do that?

Well, air likes balance. If air had its way, it would exist in the same amount at the same pressure everywhere. But this can't always be the case, so air will rush out of areas of higher pressure into areas with lower pressure in an effort to achieve balance. Think of the terrible time air has when dealing with an accordion. When the accordion is pulled apart, it creates a large space with little air in it. The air rushes in from outside the accordion (making that much-maligned accordion sound) to try to achieve balance. Then, of course, the accordionist pushes the instrument back together, creating a lot less space and more air pressure. The air forces itself out (again, making music).

A similar process occurs with breathing. When we want air to rush into our lungs, our intercostals expand the rib cage and the diaphragm flattens. This creates more space inside the chest cavity. Since air seeks a balance in pressure between the lungs and outside the body, air rushes in to fill the lungs. When we exhale, the intercostals and diaphragm return to normal, thereby shrinking the space inside our chests, and the air rushes out. When we need to blow hard, the intercostals can actually pull the ribs closer together to force even more air out.

Try it. Put your hands on your ribs just under your armpits. Now blow out until you don't have any air left. Notice how tight and pulled in your ribs feel? Now inhale normally and feel the ribs expand back out.

What does all this have to do with anxiety or relaxation? A lot, actually. When the fight-or-flight response is turned on, most of our breathing comes from the intercostals, not the diaphragm. This is because our body is trying to quickly saturate itself with oxygen for the muscles, to prepare the body to escape or fight. Fast, shallow breathing gets the oxygen in quickly and forces out a lot of carbon dioxide.

The diaphragmatic breathing exercise that follows outlines a "breathing retraining" technique that can help reduce the symptoms caused by overbreathing. It involves breathing slowly, using your diaphragm rather than your intercostal muscles. There is also a meditational component that will help you stay focused on the exercise. Note that there are different approaches to breathing retraining—this is just one variation. You may have already learned a slightly different approach during therapy, yoga classes, singing lessons, or elsewhere.

Diaphragmatic Breathing Exercise

To begin, find a spot where you can lie down comfortably on your back. Now place your left hand palm down over your belly button. Take your right hand and place it on your chest. Breathe normally through your nose. Notice how your hands are moving up and down in rhythm with your breathing. If you are relaxed right now, both hands are probably moving up and down as you breathe in and out.

Try this!

For the first part of the exercise, pretend you are walking around on a crowded beach. This means, of course, that you should suck in your belly and stick out your chest. (Don't worry—everybody does this!) Now breathe while still holding your stomach tight. Notice that only the hand on your chest is moving up and down now? This is essentially what is happening when you get anxious and begin to breathe mostly from your chest. And notice how uncomfortable this feels, and how you don't feel you're getting enough air. Does this cause you any feelings of anxiety or discomfort?

Now, allow your bottom hand to move up and down again as you breathe. Focus on your breathing, inhaling slowly and deeply so that your diaphragm gets involved and your lower hand rises. Notice how much more air you're taking in, and notice the feeling of relaxation and calmness that comes along with it. Notice how different this feels from the chest breathing. Continue breathing slowly, in and out, for 2 minutes.

For the last part of the exercise, you're going to add a component to help you focus on the exercise and increase your relaxation. Each inhalation should take about 4 seconds, as should each exhalation (if 4 seconds seems too short, you can extend the time to 5 or 6 seconds for each inhalation and each exhalation). As you inhale, mentally repeat the word "inhale" followed by the numbers 2, 3, and 4, as you count the number of seconds spent inhaling. As you exhale, mentally repeat the word "relax" followed by the numbers 2, 3, and 4, as you count the number of seconds spent exhaling. Don't hold your breath in between each inhale and exhale. Rather, keep the cycle of inhaling and exhaling smooth and relaxed.

Inhale—2—3—4

Relax—2—3—4

Inhale—2—3—4

Relax—2—3—4

Inhale—2—3—4

Relax—2—3—4

Continue the practice for about 10 minutes and do it at least twice a day.

How was that? Did you find it more or less calming than PMR?

A word of caution about breathing retraining. Although it can be a useful strategy for dealing with general anxiety, worry, tension, and stress, it should *not* be used as an avoidance strategy. If you're afraid of feeling panicky and breathless, for example, don't tell yourself, "Oh, no . . . I'm having a panic attack . . . I better slow down my breathing so I don't faint or drop dead!" This just turns breathing retraining into a safety behavior that will help your anxiety to thrive.

If you find that you're doing the breathing exercise out of fear of what might happen if you don't do it, then don't do it. (If this distinction is confusing you, please reread Chapter 8 on exposure.) But it's perfectly appropriate to use it to deal with general anxiety and stress (for example, feeling worried about all your deadlines at work, feeling stressed out by your screaming children, and so on).

Managing Stress

As discussed in Chapter 3, significant life stress can interfere with the outcome of treatment. Such stresses include health problems, relationship conflict, divorce, work stress, unemployment, financial strain, living in a dangerous neighborhood, and experiencing legal problems.

Over time, many minor stresses, such as car problems and lost luggage during a vacation, can also take their toll. Even positive life events like getting married, starting an exciting new job, or having a baby can be stressful.

There are a number of reasons why increased stress can have a negative impact on treatment. First, when we are under stress we tend to feel more emotional and vulnerable, and we experience more physical symptoms such as a racing heart, muscle tension, dizziness, and breathlessness. As a result, we're more likely to experience higher levels of fear and anxiety in situations that normally would seem manageable. For example, if you experience mild levels of fear while riding elevators, you may find that your fear of elevators is higher when you have a lot of stress at work. In addition to increasing levels of arousal, stress can affect anxiety treatment by distracting people's attention from their treatment. If you're consumed by the demands of a new baby or the threat of being laid off at work, it will be much more difficult for you to work on your OCD or your anxiety in social situations, for example.

High levels of stress can lead to a worsening of other problems as well. For example, people who get headaches tend to experience more of them when they're under stress. People who are prone to depression, anger problems, eating disorders, or alcohol abuse are at risk for having these problems worsen during or following times of stress.

As discussed in Chapter 3, if the stress you are under is temporary (for example, planning a wedding), it may be best to wait until after it has passed before beginning to work on your anxiety problem. But if your stress is ongoing (for example, raising three children and regularly lacking enough money to cover your rent and other expenses), waiting until the stress has passed may not be a realistic option. Rather, it may be best to try to deal with the stress directly.

There are two main ways of dealing with stress. The first involves trying to reduce or eliminate it, and the second involves changing the way you respond to stress.

Reducing Stress Levels

There are direct steps you can take to reduce or eliminate stress. Examples include:

- Leaving a stressful job
- Asking the boss for more flexible hours
- Reducing your college course load from five courses to four courses per semester
- Leaving an abusive relationship
- Going for marital therapy to reduce conflict in your relationship
- Getting treatment for your chronic back pain

People often respond to problems in ways that increase the stress in their lives rather than decrease it. When faced with the stress of a challenging assignment, for example, students will often put off working on it until the night before it's due, thereby compounding their stress. Postponing dealing with stress is an ineffective method of coping, particularly if the stress is unlikely to go away on its own.

Using Relaxation-Based Strategies

The relaxation exercises, including PMR and breathing retraining, are potentially helpful ways to deal with stress. The recommended readings at the back of this book contain additional resources for those who wish to learn more about these strategies.

Increasing Pleasurable Activities

Everyone needs a break from stress. If you are under a lot of stress, taking the time to do things you enjoy (for example, seeing a movie, going out with friends) is an important strategy for managing stress and reducing its impact on your health.

Healthy Lifestyle Habits

Healthy lifestyle habits are also important when dealing with stress. More than ever, it is important when under stress to eat well, seek social support, exercise, get a good night's sleep, and reduce use of caffeine, nicotine, alcohol, and other substances.

Conclusion

Relaxation-based strategies often feel great—it's no surprise that they're among the most popular techniques for treating anxiety. But they're *not* a substitute for thought challenging (Chapters 6 and 7) and exposure (Chapters 8–11). In most cases, those are the keys to overcoming anxiety. Use the relaxation skills described in this chapter to deal with general feelings of anxiety and stress, but do not rely on them exclusively as strategies for coping with more focused fears, panic attacks, OCD symptoms, and the like.

Relaxation is a skill and, like any skill, you won't get good at it unless you practice. Many people don't become completely relaxed after first trying these exercises; some get no benefit at first. Keep practicing, though—it will become easier and easier to slow down your body and mind and have one more tool at your disposal to control your anxiety.

13

mindfulness
learning to accept unwanted experiences

Mindfulness isn't a formal part of this anti-anxiety program, but if you are still struggling with anxiety or stress after having worked through the thought challenging and exposures—the core of the program—mindfulness may be another avenue that could be helpful. If you find that these mindfulness exercises are particularly helpful for you, we highly recommend *Worry Less, Live More* by Susan Orsillo and Lizabeth Roemer, and *The Mindfulness and Acceptance Workbook for Anxiety* by John Forsyth and Georg Eifert. These books are listed in the Resources.

One of the common themes you have probably gathered from this book is that trying to control your anxiety doesn't work in the long term. We talked about it in terms of trying to control or get rid of anxiety-provoking thoughts (Chapter 10) and used the example of Spotty the Bear. We talked about trying to control your anxiety by avoiding anxiety-provoking objects or situations (Chapter 9) or bodily sensations (Chapter 11). And removing your safety behaviors when doing exposures was an important focus of Chapter 8.

There is a growing recognition that instead of trying to control our anxiety-provoking thoughts, we need to do the opposite. Rather than judging, controlling, or fighting anxiety-provoking thoughts, we need to relinquish control. The power that these thoughts have comes from our reaction to them. After all, as we saw in Chapters 5–7, our anxiety-related thoughts are usually vast overestimations of the likelihood or severity of the bad things we anticipate. Learning to accept our emotions, sensations, and thoughts (versus trying to control them) is the heart of what we call mindfulness.

Mindfulness- and acceptance-based strategies are becoming increasingly popular in the treatment of anxiety problems. They can be used alongside the cognitive- and exposure-based strategies you've already learned. In fact, these more traditional strategies can be thought of as acceptance-based techniques in that they help you become more accepting of your anxiety symptoms. As we hope we've made clear by now, fighting your feelings of fear and anxiety and trying to rid yourself of scary thoughts and imagery only serve to make these symptoms worse.

Mindfulness and acceptance are not so much a set of techniques as a way to react to anxiety-related thoughts, worries, sensations, and unpleasant emotions. There are lots of different techniques for achieving a state of mindfulness and acceptance, including some of the other strategies described throughout this book. Mindfulness and acceptance emphasize the importance of *not fighting* your thoughts and feelings. After all, they are just thoughts and feelings—they're part of who you are, part of what it means to be human.

Think of it this way: Picture a scene where you are looking at a river. Imagine that your thoughts or emotions are a boat floating down the river. But you don't want the boat to block your view of the river. You could try wading into the water and holding back the boat. How effective do you think that would be? You probably would burn up a lot of energy and effort, but the boat would float along anyway. You might even slow it down slightly, which would keep it in your view even longer!

Another approach would be to get behind the boat and try to push it out of your view. Would that work? Again, probably not. You would waste a lot of time and energy without making the boat float away any faster.

Or you could allow yourself to accept that the boat is coming and that it will go away eventually. Rather than fighting the boat or getting angry about it, you could watch it come and watch it leave. You can be aware of the boat without judging it. Look at the boat. Does it have a motor or sail? How big is the boat? How deep does it sit in the water? Is there anybody on the deck of the boat?

This is the key to mindfulness and acceptance. You may not want negative emotions or anxiety-provoking thoughts, but don't fight them. Sit back, let them float along your "mental river," and let them float away. This can feel strange at first because we're so used to trying *not* to have these thoughts or feelings. But with practice, you can become an expert at letting the thoughts and emotions easily come and go. You'll be surprised by how quickly they float away when you don't fight them!

There are a number of strategies for achieving a state of mindfulness and acceptance. Some include employing images and metaphors similar to the boat metaphor; some focus on meditation. You can find some excellent books and audio recordings if you'd like to learn more about mindfulness-based meditation (see the Resources for some suggestions). Many of the strategies already described in this book (including exposure, some of the thought-challenging strategies, and relaxation) can be used to promote a state of acceptance or mindfulness.

For example, decatastrophizing (a strategy you read about in Chapter 6) helps you accept an upsetting situation or feeling, recognizing that feared outcomes are often not as bad as they seem. Similarly, imaginal exposure (Chapter 10) and interoceptive exposure (Chapter 11) teach us to be aware of and accept our uncomfortable thoughts and feelings, rather than trying to change them. So if you've been practicing these techniques, you've already been using mindfulness-based strategies even if you didn't know it. But there are some additional strategies that can help you adopt a more mindful approach, both to your anxiety-provoking thoughts and to your life.

Becoming Mindful

Mindfulness can be defined as deliberately bringing your attention to your immediate internal experiences (for example, thoughts, sensations, emotions) and attending to them compassionately and nonjudgmentally. Mindfulness involves being in the present moment, rather than worrying about the future or dwelling on the past. It involves just being with your thoughts and your experiences—without judging them or trying to change or control them. This can sometimes be difficult at first for people who have had problems with anxiety or depression because these experiences can feel unpleasant, but it is something that most people can achieve with practice.

The following three exercises are designed to help you develop your ability to become and stay mindful of the moment. They don't deal directly with your anxiety—we'll get to that later. Rather, they are intentionally *not* about your anxiety-related thoughts, so that you can develop your mindfulness skills more generally before turning to your anxiety. Try each of these exercises one at a time and practice that one every day for a week. Then try another one the next week, until you have had a chance to thoroughly practice all three.

> **Mindfulness Exercises**
> - **Mindful eating**
> - **Mindful listening**
> - **Mindful body scan**

1. Mindful Eating Exercise

A popular exercise for introducing people to mindfulness involves examining a raisin, but really any food will work. Right now, I (Peter) have a banana with me as I type this. The objective is to explore the piece of food in all of its aspects without judgment. Let it sit on the plate in front of you and look at it. What color is it? Is it all the same color, or are there variations? Is it shiny and reflective, or does it have more of a matte finish? My banana is mostly yellow but is slightly green near each end. It also has very tiny light-brown dots on it, especially on the inside of the curve. I see a small dent in the skin of the banana that is a darker shade of brown. Part of the stem is exposed, and I can see the coarse fibers of the stem.

Now touch the piece of food. Pick it up and put it in your hand. Gently roll it around in your fingers. What does it feel like? What words would you use to describe its texture? Is it firm or soft? My banana feels firm to the touch. The skin has a waxy feel and is smooth to the touch. I feel ridges along the skin of the banana; I had never noticed those before. The bottom tip of the banana has a rough texture, and is a much darker brown than anywhere else on the banana.

Before you taste the piece of food, try to experience it in different ways first. Does it have a smell? Do different parts of it smell the same way? When you gently tap it, does it make a sound?

What is my experience of this food?

I'm not getting any smell from the outside of my banana, but it makes a soft hollow sound like a little drum when I gently tap the skin. As I start to peel the banana it makes a crackling sound when it first breaks and then a soft tearing sound as it peels back along the ridges I felt earlier.

Now put the piece of food in your mouth, but don't chew or swallow it yet. How does it feel in your mouth? Sit with the experience of holding it on your tongue. What tastes are you experiencing?

What textures? Does it change as you hold it in your mouth? Now after a minute or two, take a single bite. How has it changed? Is the flavor different? The texture? The experience? Chew it some more. What are you experiencing now? Eventually, once you have chewed the food, allow yourself to swallow the food and experience the feeling of it sliding down your throat.

2. Mindful Listening Exercise

For your next practice, put yourself in a place where you can be alone and comfortable for 15 minutes. This can be anywhere that you won't be interrupted—in the bathtub, under a tree in the backyard, on the sofa in your living room, or on a bench at the park. Once you are comfortable, start by listening to your own breathing. Take a long slow inhale, hold it for a second, and then exhale. Listen to and experience the sounds of the air entering and leaving your lungs. If you find yourself judging the experience—perhaps you heard a wheeze—just try to put those thoughts aside and refocus your attention on the sounds and experiences.

Now expand your focus to the sounds around you. Notice the different sounds. Do some of them come and go? Are some of the more constant? How loud or soft are the different sounds? Do they have different pitches, like different notes from a musical instrument? Try to push your attention even farther out. Can you hear traffic in the distance? Perhaps you can hear the air blowing out of the vents. Are there any conversations going on or music playing? Remember to listen and experience the sounds without judgment. If you find a sound to be irritating or aversive, gently put that judgement aside and just try to listen and experience the sounds.

After about 15 minutes, allow your focus to come back to you. What were some of the sounds you heard? Maybe some of the sounds came from you, like your breathing or a gurgle in your stomach. Perhaps you heard sounds nearby, like the leaves rustling when the wind blew or a drip from the bathtub faucet. Maybe they were far away, like an airplane in the distance or a dog barking. What were the sounds like? Were you able to keep your mind on the experience rather than judging the sounds?

What is my experience with the sounds?

3. Mindful Body Scan

The third exercise is similar to the previous two, but instead of engaging in a nonjudgmental experience of things external to you—like the food or the sounds—you're going to do the same with your body. This exercise can be a little more difficult at first because many of us have things about our body (for example, aspects of our appearance, bodily sensations, or physical health problems) that we don't like. This can make it difficult to attend to and experience these things in a nonjudgmental way. But this is also why this exercise can be so helpful to keep practicing. For if we can learn to nonjudgmentally attend to aspects of our selves that we're least fond of, then we can probably develop the ability to be mindful about anything.

Find a place where you can comfortably lie back and not be disturbed for the next 30 minutes. We would recommend not doing this in bed at first, as that could make it too easy to fall asleep. Once you are comfortable, close your eyes and attend to your own breathing. Pay attention to the feelings of your chest and stomach rising and falling as you bring the air into and out of your lungs. Pay attention to any other feelings or sensations you have. Again, if you notice yourself evaluating or judging, gently put those thoughts aside and try to immerse yourself in the experience of breathing.

Now, while still attending to your breathing, let your attention expand to the feelings in your toes and feet. What sensations do you feel? What is the experience of attending to your toes and feet? When you feel ready, slowly move your attention to your lower legs and go through the same experience. Then to your knees, then thighs. Continue in this way up your body, stopping at the hips and pelvis, your stomach and lower back, chest, shoulders, upper arms, lower arms, and hands and fingers. When you have reached your fingers, come back up to your neck, then your head. Remember, at each stop along your body, try to attend to the feelings and parts of your body without judgment. As you did with the piece of food or the sounds, try to immerse yourself in the experience of each part of your body. If your mind gets drawn elsewhere, or if you find yourself evaluating or judging some part of your bodily experience, that's okay. Just redirect your attention to simply experiencing that part of your body.

What is my experience with these feelings?

Bindi—Mindfully Staying Present

Bindi, the socially anxious university student, really liked the concept of mindfulness as it sounded very similar to some of the cultural practices the elders of her clan had taught her about when she was younger. In particular, she was very attracted to the idea of mindful listening as a way of reconnecting with the world around her. She was feeling a bit disconnected from nature, being on a large university campus in the big city. So Bindi took her book to a large wooded park nearby, reread the instructions, and practiced mindful listening. As she practiced extending her awareness, she was able to hear the breeze blowing through the leaves of the trees and a number of bird calls—some of which she had never heard before. She also could hear some traffic from a highway in the distance, which she initially didn't like, but she practiced accepting those sounds nonjudgmentally. She recognized that all of these sounds had a place together as part of a larger whole. As she continued to practice mindful listening every few days, she found that she was able to achieve a centered and mindful feeling more easily in other areas of her life, such as when she was worried about exams or when the neighbors in her dorm were making noise late at night. She also found that she was able to allow herself to accept her feelings of homesickness. "I am allowed to miss my family and friends; that just means that I love them and enjoy their company. Right now I am on another journey, and I will be able to see them again," she would remind herself.

Becoming Mindful of Your Anxiety-Provoking Thoughts

The point of the three exercises on pages 210–212 is to demonstrate how we often go through life on autopilot, rather than consciously and purposely experiencing the moment. When we're not present in the moment, we tend to act or react without thought. Rather than simply reacting to thoughts and situations, take the time to consciously, deliberately, and nonjudgmentally experience them. Experience them for what they are, rather than what you expect or want them to be.

Approaching your anxiety-provoking thoughts and worries is done in a very similar way. The first step, which you have already practiced, is to become aware of your thoughts. When you have a thought such as "Bad things are going to happen to me" or "Everyone will think I'm stupid," rather than push it away or react to it, try to hold on to it and examine it nonjudgmentally. Be like an archaeologist who has just found a new artifact and examine it without judgment or preconceived expectations. Acknowledge that the thought is just a thought, not a reality.

Next, try to distance yourself from the thought. See the thought as just a thought and label it as such: "I am having a thought that everyone will think I'm stupid" instead of "Everyone will think I'm stupid." Identify what type of anxious thought it is (from back in Chapter 5): "I am having a probability-overestimation thought that everyone will think I'm stupid."

Once you have distanced yourself from that thought, try to defuse the power of that thought. Play around with the thought by saying it out loud in different voices or accents. Picture it written out in different fonts: *I am having* a probability-overestimation thought **that everyone will think I'm stupid.** The goal here is to defuse the emotional power of the thought by distancing yourself from what the thought is trying to tell you. Is it something that still makes you anxious? If so, acknowledge that. *I am feeling anxious because I am having a probability-overestimation thought that everyone will think I'm stupid.* A thought is just a thought—not a reality. An emotion is just an emotion—not a reality.

An important thing to note, however, is that being mindful and nonjudgmental with your thoughts and experiences is *not* the same as giving in or resigning yourself to those thoughts or experiences. Giving in or resigning yourself would be like saying, "I'll never get any better so there is no point trying," while someone being mindful and nonjudgmental would say, "I am feeling anxious about this right now, and that is okay." Do you notice the difference? Resignation is more of a sense of helplessness and hopelessness, while mindfulness is accepting what you are feeling or thinking without fighting those thoughts or feelings.

Conclusion

Mindfulness is becoming a very popular approach for dealing with anxiety and depression. The research evidence supporting mindful approaches is not quite as established as it is for other cognitive and behavioral approaches, but it is highly promising. In fact, many mental health professionals have questioned whether the skills and techniques of mindfulness and CBT are really that different. Even so, if you find that this approach is working well for you, we strongly encourage you to continue practicing the techniques.

The three exercises we recommended, mindful eating, mindful listening, and mindful body scanning, are excellent ways to help train yourself to adopt a mindful mindset and begin to mindfully and nonjudgmentally acknowledge and view your anxious thinking. But, like everything else in this book (and in life!), becoming more mindful is a skill that must be practiced. Set aside time every day to work through these exercises, but also take opportunities to allow yourself to practice these skills informally—while you are in the shower, when you are slicing vegetables for dinner, or when you are walking to the bus stop.

conclusion
living without anxiety

You should read this chapter once you have tamed your anxiety problem. For example, when you are no longer avoiding the things you used to avoid because of anxiety or fear, when your panic attacks are much less frequent, or when you no longer experience intense fear if you encounter the things that used to frighten you, it is probably time to delve into this chapter. This chapter will help you develop the skills to keep your anxiety problem away as you shift from *fighting against it* toward *living without it*. However, even if your anxiety problem isn't where you would like it to be yet, this chapter will also provide strategies for identifying which chapters and sections you should go back to and keep working on.

Where Is Your Anxiety Now?

At the beginning of this book, you spent a fair amount of time examining your anxiety and rating how much it affected you and your life. Now that your anxiety has improved, you should go through those steps again, for two reasons:

1. **Seeing how much you have improved can motivate you to maintain those gains.** Few things are as powerful as previous success for increasing your motivation to keep up your hard work. When you see how far you've come, you'll want to protect those improvements and do whatever you can to prevent a return of your anxiety.

2. **Reassessing your anxiety can help you identify areas that are still causing difficulty.** On occasion, when people have made great gains in overcoming their anxiety in most areas of their life, they focus on those improvements while ignoring areas that still cause problems. This can lead to difficulties later because the more leftover symptoms you have now, the more likely the anxiety can creep back and start to take over your life again.

In Chapter 2, you described several aspects of your anxiety and rated how severe they were. Flip back to that chapter (or pull out the forms if you downloaded them) and remind yourself of what you wrote in Forms 2.4 (Thoughts Associated with My Anxiety Problems), 2.5 (Situations I Avoid), 2.6 (My Safety Behaviors), and 2.7 (Fear of Physical Sensations). Notice the ratings that you gave on each form. Now go ahead and rerate each of these based on how you are feeling *right now*. Now that you have worked through the program, how much change have you experienced?

Look over these lists and ratings and compare how you felt when you started this workbook to how you feel now. Have you made the gains you had hoped to? Are you able to do things you couldn't do before? Have you been able to control and change your anxiety-provoking thinking? Were you able to give up your safety behaviors and face your anxiety head on? For every achievement you've made, you should congratulate yourself. It required hard work, courage, and determination. Congratulations!

You deserve a reward or celebration, even if you are not 100% happy with the reduction in your anxiety problem. Even a moderate reduction is something worth celebrating. Go out for dinner and a movie. Or stay in and cook a nice dinner and stream a movie. Go dancing. Send your kids to their grandparents' house for the night.

While patting yourself on the back for the gains you've made, you might also feel that you still have some goals you haven't reached. Are there areas where you feel you need to keep working? If so, go back to Chapters 5–7 to review how you can use thought challenging to confront those remaining negative thoughts, and Chapters 8–11 to continue confronting the situations, thoughts, or physical sensations that continue to provoke your anxiety. Don't worry; this chapter will still be here once you get the remainder of your anxiety problems under control.

I'm Happy with My Improvement—What Now?

> **Anti-Anxiety Toolkit**
> **Challenging your thoughts**
> **Exposure**
> **Relaxation**
> **Mindfulness**

If you genuinely believe that you have your anxiety problems under control, then now is the time to shift from *making your gains* to *maintaining your gains*. This doesn't mean closing this book and never thinking about your anxiety again. Even if you believe that you're "cured," anxiety problems can be sneaky and find their way back into your life. Even world-class pianists need to practice scales every now and then, and pro golfers need to keep practicing at the driving range. Similarly, you must practice your anti-anxiety skills periodically to maintain your gains.

A first step is to review which strategies had the biggest impact on your anxiety. For many people, especially those who fear specific situations, objects, activities, thoughts, or sensations, that would be the exposure exercises. Others find greater success with the thought-challenging or relaxation skills. Write down those skills that you feel were most important in your recovery:

1. _____

2. _____

3. _____

Now start to develop a plan to work these strategies into your regular routine. We strongly encourage you to continue practicing these skills. You probably don't need to spend as much time practicing as you did while working through the earlier chapters, but please don't stop! As with anything you've worked to master, you'll lose the skill if you don't keep it alive.

Keeping Up Your Anti-Anxiety Skills

Jamal was a former patient who went through this program because of his intense fears of public speaking and social interactions. He had even refused a promotion at work (and a substantial pay raise) because he was terrified of having to make occasional presentations to the board and to manage the people working under him. During his treatment, he practiced communicating assertively and confidently with his coworkers. He also practiced talking to small audiences.

As he continued his treatment, Jamal started to practice giving presentations to larger and larger audiences. By the time he was finished, he felt very little anxiety when standing up and talking in front of others. He was able to accept the promotion and found that he was more than capable of presenting to the board and managing his department.

But Jamal was wise enough to realize that he needed to continue to work on his anti-anxiety skills. After finishing the program, he joined a local chapter of Toastmasters International. For a small fee, members get together regularly to give talks, presentations, and speeches to improve their speaking skills. Jamal decided to attend these meetings once a month to help him stay on top of his improvements. He also joined the board of his homeowners' association so that he would have opportunities to practice being assertive. Both of these activities were a great help to him in maintaining his improvements.

What about you? What are some activities you could do every now and then to keep your anti-anxiety skills fresh? You don't need to do them daily or even weekly. Here are some examples:

Former Fears	Current Activities
Certain animals	About once a month, go to the zoo, humane society, or other places where you're likely to see your previously feared animal.
Bodily sensations	Every 2 weeks, practice the interoceptive exposure exercises that you found most helpful in Chapter 11.
Social fears	Join groups where you can interact with people. Ask your boss for an opportunity to present at meetings occasionally.

Former Fears	Current Activities
Contamination fears	Each month, for one afternoon, make a point of going out and touching things that used to concern you.
Worries about your family's safety	If you previously tended to use your cell phone to seek reassurance that your family members are safe, pick a day that is going to be your "no cell phone" day. Go out for the day and practice keeping your worries at bay.

Now, think of what you could do to maintain your gains. Write these ideas down on Conclusion Form 1 and post this list somewhere you will see it and be reminded to keep up your practice. (The form provides space for three fears; if you need more space, photocopy the form or download and print extra copies; see the end of the Contents for information.)

Predicting and Recovering from Lapses and Relapses

Now for the inevitable reminder: setbacks happen. Many, if not most, people going through this program will have a lapse at some point in the first year or two, especially during times of stress.

But a *lapse* isn't the same as a *relapse*. A *lapse* is a temporary setback in which you experience a return of symptoms or you stop using the skills you learned. You may find yourself avoiding something you should be doing, cleaning something that doesn't really need cleaning, having a panic attack after several panic-free months, triple-checking something when you should trust yourself, worrying excessively about something minor, and so on. Lapses can happen after a bad experience—after a person who used to fear flying has a bumpy flight or a person who had contamination fears comes down with the flu—or they can happen for no obvious reason.

A *relapse,* on the other hand, is a more severe setback, in which your anxiety returns with full force, taking control over some part of your life again, sometimes taking you back to square one.

Dealing with Lapses

If you experience a lapse, try not to get worked up over it. You have the skills to get yourself back on track. Practice challenging your anxiety-provoking thoughts. Perform your own exposures to get your fears back under control.

The funny thing about lapses is that, in hindsight, you might possibly have seen them coming. Lapses usually happen when we're under stress or in a difficult situation. For some, going back to classes after the summer break is a time when they're prone to lapses. Others find that even pleasant times, such as the holiday season or preparing for a vacation, can put them at risk of a lapse.

What about you? Are there times when you feel you might be at greater risk of a lapse or setback? Think about it and make a list on page 220.

Strategies for Maintaining Gains

My former fears	My activities for keeping the anxiety away for good
Fear 1	
Fear 2	
Fear 3	

_____

_____

_____

_____

_____

If you know there are times when you might be prone to a lapse, you can prepare yourself in advance. Perhaps you can open up Chapter 12 and practice relaxation exercises. Maybe you can increase how often you practice those skills you decided you would use to maintain your gains. Maybe you can prepare for stressful situations so they're a little less stressful. Take some time to generate some ideas you can use to prepare for situations where you're at risk for a lapse and then write them down:

_____

_____

_____

_____

Dealing with Relapses

As much as we hope they won't, relapses sometimes happen. Sometimes lapses build up unexpectedly and you find yourself returning to your old anxious patterns. This can feel very discouraging. People often "beat themselves up" for letting that happen.

Rather than punishing yourself for a relapse, take control and remind yourself that you beat the anxiety once before—you can do it again! This time it will be even easier to gain control over your anxiety because you already know what to do. Go back through this program and work through the exercises that helped you previously. Challenge your negative thoughts and expose yourself to your anxiety triggers again. Resume your relaxation exercises, if these were helpful previously. Look at your lifestyle habits to see if there are areas you can improve. By resuming the strategies that were helpful before, you will regain your control over your anxiety.

What are some signs that you might be having a relapse instead of simply a lapse? Janet previously had agoraphobia and didn't leave her home for fear that she might have a panic attack. She worked through this program and overcame her fears. She now goes out to malls and crowded places with very little anxiety. But she knows that old habits sometimes have a way of coming back, so she identified several warning signs to alert herself that a relapse might be coming on. She then developed a plan to get back in control of her anxiety (see Sample Completed Conclusion Form 2).

What are your own signs that you might be starting to relapse? Write them down on Conclusion Form 2 and develop your own plan for regaining control. Keep this sheet handy so that at the first sign of trouble you will know what you need to do. (If you need extra space,

SAMPLE COMPLETED CONCLUSION FORM 2 *(Janet)*

My Plan for Dealing with Relapses

Signs of relapse	My action plan to get back my control
I go four straight days without leaving the house.	*Immediately pull out this book and challenge my anxious thoughts.*
	Get dressed and go to the mall right away to practice my exposures. Do this every day for a week.
I start freaking out about funny sensations in my body.	*Immediately pull out this book and challenge my anxious thoughts that something might be wrong with me.*
	Reread Chapter 11 and start practicing the exposures to bodily sensations twice a day for 2 weeks.

photocopy or download and print additional sheets; see the end of the Contents for information about downloading.)

Moving On

Though it's important to understand that setbacks can happen and to prepare yourself to cope with possible triggers for relapse, you need to focus on what's most important—*the improvements you have made in overcoming your anxiety and taking back your life.*

Using the space below and on page 223, you need to do a couple more exercises—and then you'll be done with all the forms in this program! First, write down the most important things you can do now that you couldn't do before because of your anxiety.

1. _____

   _____

My Plan for Dealing with Relapses

Signs of a relapse	My action plan to get back my control

2. _____

_____

3. _____

_____

4. _____

_____

5. _____

_____

To reward myself, what would I like to do that anxiety prevented me from doing?

Doesn't it feel spectacular to be able to do these things again (or for the first time)?

Now, write down at least three things that you are *going to do* in the near future that you were prevented from doing because of your anxiety. Maybe take that vacation you avoided because of your fears of flying or driving. Or make the big purchase you put off because of unrealistic financial worries. It even could involve signing up for a dating or singles club now that you've overcome your social fears. What do you want to achieve now that you can?

1. _____

_____

2. _____

_____

3. _____

_____

4. _____

_____

5. _____

_____

Now pick one (or more!), and go ahead and do it. You've earned it!

Epilogue: Success Stories

Valerie

Valerie's mind was always coming up with things to worry about. Before she started the program, she was anxious all the time about all sorts of things, but often the worries were tied to the safety of her husband, Carl, and the strength of their marriage. In fact, she even worried that her worries would cause Carl to get tired of her and leave. Valerie was very motivated to reduce her worries and anxiety, but, of course, she was worried that the program wouldn't work for her. Even so, she really committed herself to the program, thinking to herself, "If I really give it a good try, at best I'll be a calm and relaxed person; at worst, all I will have lost is some time reading a book and doing the exercises."

After reading the first few chapters and assessing her own form of anxiety, she was very interested in the cognitive strategies that were going to come up in Chapters 5, 6, and 7, as well as the relaxation skills in Chapter 12. She also realized that she would probably have to do the cognitive exposure exercises in Chapter 10. She wasn't too keen on the idea of exposures, but felt that she needed to do everything she could to beat her worries.

Personally, Valerie didn't find the thought-challenging exercises to be as helpful at first as she had hoped. She understood the rationale and logic, but she didn't believe the rational responses. After all, people had been telling her that her worries were unrealistic for years. Even so, she hung on to her motivation and started the exposures. After reading Chapter 8 and developing her hierarchy, she knew that she would need to go all in with the exposures in Chapter 10. She didn't really have any specific situations or bodily sensations that caused her anxiety to spike; it was always these thoughts that would start her into what she called a "worry spiral."

In Chapter 10, we described one of her most powerful worry exposures. It was the one where she made a worry script about her husband cheating on her. That was one of her more common worries, even though there was no evidence that he had done, or would do, such a thing. Feel free to go back and read her experience with this exposure. Given how much her worries about this decreased over the next days and weeks, she wrote out several more worry scripts and repeated the process. One was about Carl being in a car accident on his drive in to work. Another was on her worries that tensions between the government and other countries might escalate into a full-scale war. Each time, it would take her a few days of reading and rereading her worry script, but each time her anxiety and worries would start to dissipate. In fact, she started to notice that other worries about which she hadn't done an exposure were also going down. She was retraining her brain not to get caught up in her "worry spirals"!

When Valerie got to Chapter 12, she hated the breathing retraining. She found that just breathing actually gave her brain time to start trying to come up with new worries. On the other hand, she loved the progressive muscle relaxation (PMR). She liked doing things, and the focus on her muscle tension and relaxation was right up her alley. With practice, Valerie got to the point where she could do the full-body PMR from memory and was able to get herself into a highly relaxed state very easily. She avoided doing the PMR when she was working on her worry script exposures but found that practicing PMR first thing in the morning and later in the evening was a great way to start and end her day. And she felt that it was a much better and healthier way of relaxing her body than having a gin and tonic.

Valerie was also very intrigued about the idea of mindfulness in Chapter 13. She had heard about mindfulness but never knew what it involved. She found the exercises enjoyable and calming and decided that she would order one of the recommended books . . . although she hasn't actually gotten around to reading it yet because she was already feeling so much less anxious and worried.

To reward herself, Valerie decided that she and Carl should go on a vacation. They hadn't been on one in many years, mostly because of her worries. She would worry about picking the wrong vacation spot, messing up the airplane and hotel reservations, that something would happen to their home while away . . . you get the idea. So she did a few extra worry exposures about these things and then started to plan the vacation. She organized everything without seeking reassurance from Carl, and the two of them spent an incredibly relaxing week on a tropical cruise. And when Carl went on a scuba dive excursion—she couldn't go because of problems with her ears when going underwater—she didn't let herself get caught up in worries about him drowning or getting eaten by sharks. She was too busy working on her suntan!

Jacob

Jacob was the man who, when he was younger, saw his father have a stroke. As he got older, he began having panic attacks any time he felt a headache coming on.

Jacob decided to read the whole book first before jumping in and doing the exercises. The first thing Jacob did after reading the book was make a commitment to himself to stop going to the hospital every time he had a headache. He understood how these coping behaviors were keeping his anxiety strong, and he also was getting frustrated at how much the emergency room visits were costing.

The cognitive skills he learned and practiced in Chapters 5, 6, and 7 were a revelation to him. He had never seriously considered any possibility for headaches other than "it's a stroke!" He actually felt kind of silly when he started to generate alternate possibilities for a headache. "I have a stressful job, work long hours, and I drink a lot of coffee." These skills really helped him quickly interrupt the automatic assumption that he was having a stroke, which stopped the escalation into a panic attack. (He also decided to cut back on his coffee drinking and make some changes in how much extra work he took on.)

Next, Jacob started working on doing the interoceptive exposures in Chapter 11. He found that some of the exercises created strong sensations in his body, such as lightheadedness from spinning in a chair. But Jacob understood the concept and designed a few interoceptive exposure exercises that did work. He found that staring intensely at himself in the mirror would give him a bit of a headache, which worked well for the exposure. He also would tie a headband tightly around his head (he thought he looked like the character from the Rambo movies), and this really created strong headache-like sensations, which caused his anxiety to spike quickly. As he practiced these exposures over and over again, he quickly found that his anxiety each time wouldn't go up as high as the previous time, although a brief bout of the flu did cause him some minor setbacks where he worried a lot about his health. But once he started feeling healthier again, he restarted his exposures. And after he did these exercises for a few weeks, the sensations no longer scared him.

So Jacob decided to do a traumatic memory script like the one in Chapter 10 for the memory of his father having a stroke in front of him. He had tried to avoid thinking about it for so long, which told him that an exposure would probably be a good idea. He wrote out the script, which was very anxiety provoking for him, and then recorded himself reading it using his phone. His anxiety level was pretty high when he read the script into the phone, but not as bad as when he was writing it. It was quite emotional for him, though, as he hadn't really thought about that day in detail in a long time. Nonetheless, by the time he started listening to the recording he found that it wasn't causing him much distress anymore. After a few days of listening to it, the memory no longer caused him any anxiety, just some sadness for what his father had experienced.

The relaxation and mindfulness chapters didn't do much for Jacob. He wasn't really anxious or tense most of the time. His anxiety was almost always tied to headaches. When he got to this chapter, he had some trouble coming up with ways he could reward himself that would be tied to his previous fears and panic attacks. But he decided that since he was much more comfortable with the bodily sensations and he wasn't having panic attacks anymore, he really wanted to start getting back in shape. He hadn't exercised in a long time, so he decided to join a gym and start meeting up with people to go running. Jacob hadn't had a partner or many dates in a while. Partly this was because of his panic and fears, but he also didn't feel that other men would find him very attractive since he hadn't worked out in so long. So he decided that rewarding himself by starting to exercise again could lead to even better rewards down the road.

Bindi

Having moved from her traditional lands to attend a university in a large city, Bindi became very socially anxious and withdrawn. She also started to feel depressed, probably because she was staying in her apartment all the time and not socializing and had begun to have occasional scary thoughts of not wanting to be alive. In Chapter 9, we gave a very detailed account of the exposures she did to help her overcome her social anxiety. With guidance from a psychologist, she started by just talking to a couple of classmates every day, then asking or answering questions in class. And then she started having dinner or coffee with a classmate she was becoming good friends with. After a while, she started pushing herself by joining an Indigenous Students' Association group on campus, which led to opportunities to give presentations and even to a date.

Bindi found that the exercises in the chapter on relaxation felt nice but didn't really do anything for her anxiety. She was already beating her anxiety through exposures. But she quite enjoyed the exercises in the chapter on mindfulness, as many of the concepts seemed to coincide with some of her community's cultural beliefs. She found these exercises particularly helpful in dealing with her feelings of homesickness and cultural isolation, but also in not beating herself up emotionally when she did have thoughts of being judged or not fitting in.

Finally, Bindi spent a lot of time going over the sections in this chapter on dealing with lapses and relapses. Although she was doing really well, she felt like her social doubts could easily creep back into her life unless she was vigilant about continuing to develop, practice, and expand her social activities. She never wanted to isolate herself again and have thoughts that life wasn't worth living. Around this time, Bindi and her psychologist decided to suspend their weekly sessions, as Bindi was doing so well. To this day, Bindi continues to assign herself weekly exposure goals. They aren't always "big deal" exposures, but she makes a firm commitment to try something different every week.

Bindi did feel a bit silly about rewarding herself for overcoming her social anxiety, and as a student she didn't have much money to do anything big. But her new friend Lynn came up with a fantastic idea. During the semester break they would go on a road trip together and stay for a few days back in Bindi's home community. Bindi loved this. She had been longing to go home for a visit, she could introduce Lynn to her family and community, and it would also be like another big exposure in that she had never spent that much consecutive time with anybody except her family. At last report, the trip had been great fun for everyone, and Bindi was very grateful to have had the chance to return to her lands and be with her family.

Jacqui

Jacqui was the woman who had terrifying intrusive thoughts of harming her newborn child, and would likely be diagnosed with a form of postnatal obsessive–compulsive disorder (OCD). She would never have actually done anything to harm her daughter, but these thoughts were so distressing that she feared they meant that she was a horrible person who *might* do something terrible. So she tried to do everything she could to get rid of the thoughts.

Jacqui chose to work through the program with a therapist who specialized in cognitive-behavioral therapy (or CBT), from which this program is derived. Jacqui was hesitant about the idea of automatic thoughts (Chapter 5) and thought challenging (Chapter 6) but had a break-through with the cognitive experiments described in Chapter 7. Simply evaluating the evidence didn't seem to change her assumptions about her intrusive thoughts, but Jacqui and her therapist set up a survey (described in more detail in Chapter 7) that really helped her test her belief that the thoughts meant she was a bad mom and she *would* harm her baby. She anonymously posted her survey question on an online new moms' forum. To her surprise, she found out that a great many moms had similar thoughts every now and then, which helped Jacqui realize that she isn't a horrible person for having these kinds of thoughts. This gave Jacqui the confidence and trust in herself to engage in the exposures described in Chapter 9, where she became comfortable leaving her daughter with her in-laws or driving on the freeway with her child in the car. She also engaged in several of the cognitive exposures in Chapter 10. In particular, rather than trying to avoid or negate the intrusive thoughts, she would try to force those thoughts into her mind repeatedly until they no longer caused her great distress. In fact, nearing the end of treatment, she remarked how "a thought is just a thought; it isn't a desire, it isn't a premonition, and it doesn't have any meaning." And as the intrusive thoughts began to lose their power over her, Jacqui noticed that they came into her mind much less frequently, if at all.

As mentioned at the end of the Introduction, Jacqui and her partner have since had another child, a healthy baby boy, and are thinking about a third. Four years on from her experience with anxiety and intrusive thoughts, Jacqui rarely has any more intrusive thoughts like these. On the rare occasion when she does, she accepts that it is "just one of those stupid thoughts" and carries on.

You

What is your story of success with the program? What parts did you find most beneficial? Did you achieve your goals? Have you been able to maintain those goals or get back on the path if you have had any lapses? We certainly hope so, and we sincerely wish you a future without anxiety.

resources

This list of helpful resources includes therapy referrals (in and outside the United States), online resources, digital tools and apps, and recommended books on a range of anxiety-related topics.

Therapy Referrals in the United States

Though based in the United States, most of these associations offer details for finding therapists and other resources both in the United States and Canada, and several offer information on resources in other countries.

Academy of Cognitive and Behavioral Therapies (Academy of CBT)
http://academyofct.org
• Website offers therapy referrals to academy-certified CBT therapists.

American Psychological Association
http://apa.org
• Website includes a section for finding a psychologist (*http://locator.apa.org*).

Anxiety and Depression Association of America (ADAA)
http://adaa.org
• In addition to a find-a-therapist section, the website contains numerous resources for consumers, including an online community; information on support groups in the United States, Canada, Australia, and South Africa; and information on mobile apps.

Association for Behavioral and Cognitive Therapies (ABCT)
http://abct.org
• Website includes a Find-a-Therapist section, *http://www.findcbt.org*.

International OCD Foundation (IOCDF)
http://iocdf.org
• In addition to providing information on professionals in the United States, Canada, and elsewhere who treat OCD, this association also has an annual conference.

Referrals Outside the United States

Anxiety Canada

http://anxietycanada.com

• In addition to information about referrals in Canada, this website includes access to a variety of other resources, including information about anxiety and its popular mobile app, MindShift CBT.

British Association for Behavioural and Cognitive Psychotherapies (BABCP)

http://babcp.com

• Website includes a "find-a-therapist" feature for individuals in the United Kingdom.

Canadian Association of Cognitive and Behavioural Therapies

http://cacbt.ca

• Website provides a list of CACBT-certified therapists in Canada.

European Association for Behavioural and Cognitive Therapies

http://eabct.eu

• Website includes a "find-a-therapist" section for CBT therapists throughout Europe (*http://eabct.eu/find-a-therapist*).

Online Resources and Information

Although the information in this section was up to date when this book went to press, web pages come and go, and addresses for Internet resources change frequently. For additional information on Internet resources, we suggest doing a search using keywords such as *anxiety, anxiety disorder, panic disorder, social anxiety, phobia, obsessive–compulsive disorder, posttraumatic stress disorder,* and so on. Note that although we have screened each of these sites, we have not reviewed them in detail, and cannot take responsibility for the accuracy of the information they contain.

Anxieties.com

http://anxieties.com

• A very informative anxiety self-help site run by Dr. Reid Wilson and the Anxiety Disorders Treatment Center in Durham, North Carolina

Anxiety Treatment Australia

http://anxietyaustralia.com.au

• A website that provides information about treatment options in Australia. The site also includes a comprehensive list of helpful resources, including websites (*www.anxietyaustralia.com.au/resources*)

Freedom from Fear

http://freedomfromfear.org

• National nonprofit advocacy organization for people with anxiety disorders and depression

• Newsletter, blogs, bookstore

• Information on support groups and other resources

Internet Mental Health

http://mentalhealth.com

- Comprehensive website with information on mental health issues

National Alliance on Mental Illness

http://nami.org

- Provides comprehensive resources on a wide range of mental health issues

National Center for PTSD

www.ptsd.va.gov

- Provides information on PTSD and its treatment

NIMH Anxiety Disorders Website

www.nimh.nih.gov/health/topics/anxiety-disorders/index.shtml

- Up-to-date information about anxiety disorders and their treatment

Parenting Strategies/Therapist-Assisted Online Parenting Strategies (TOPS)

http://parentingstrategies.net

http://tops.partnersinparenting.net.au

- Online resources and therapist-assisted online program for parents of children with depression and anxiety

Sidran Institute

http://sidran.org

- Provides information, education, and advocacy for issues related to traumatic stress

Social Anxiety Association

http://socialphobia.org

- Site for a nonprofit organization focused on social phobia and social anxiety

Social Phobia World

http://socialphobiaworld.com

- A place for online forums and chats about social phobia

Digital Tools and Apps

In this section, we review several online treatments and digital apps for tracking progress and working through CBT strategies. For information on these and other mobile apps, check out the reviews on PsyberGuide (*http://psyberguide.org*). PsyberGuide evaluates not only usability and overall experience, but also privacy and transparency, and the credibility of the research behind each app.

MindShift CBT (free; *www.anxietycanada.com/resources/mindshift-cbt*) is a digital mobile app designed to help teens and young adults manage their anxiety. It includes strategies for a wide range of anxiety problems, including social anxiety. App available for Android and iOS.

MoodKit (under $10; *http://thriveport.com*) offers a component to rate your mood and track your progress over time, providing nice digital graphs of changes in your mood. At this time, Mood-Kit is available for iOS only, but an Android version is being developed.

MoodMission (free, offers in-app purchases; *http://moodmission.com*) is an evidence-based app designed for depression and anxiety self-help.

Sanvello for Stress & Anxiety (free, but with optional in-app purchases; *http://sanvello.com/self-care*) allows users to make a single daily rating of their mood and displays a graph of changes over the week.

Self-Help for Anxiety Management (free; *http://sam-app.org.uk*) allows users to rate their feelings of anxiety and tension, unpleasant physical sensations, worrying thoughts, and avoidance using simple slide bars. The app then shows colorful graphs to help you monitor your progress over time in each of these areas.

This Way Up (costs associated; *https://thiswayup.org.au*) provides evidence-based Internet self-help treatment programs for anxiety and depression.

Way Forward (costs associated; *https://wayforward.io*) provides an online program providing either self-help or coach-assisted treatment for social anxiety using cognitive-behavioral techniques. Fees depend on the level of coach involvement.

Recommended Books

The list below includes self-help publications on CBT, relaxation, acceptance, and meditation.

Anxiety and Related Topics (General)

Alberti, R., & Emmons, M. (2017). *Your perfect right* (10th ed.). Oakland, CA: New Harbinger.

Carney, C. C., & Manber, R. (2009). *Quiet your mind and get to sleep.* Oakland, CA: New Harbinger.

Clark, D. A., & Beck, A. T. (2012). *The anxiety and worry workbook: The cognitive-behavioral solution.* New York: Guilford Press.

Davis, M., Eshelman, A. R., & McKay, M. (2019). *The relaxation and stress reduction workbook* (7th ed.). Oakland, CA: New Harbinger.

Forsyth, G., & Eifert, G. (2016). *The mindfulness and acceptance workbook for anxiety* (2nd ed.). Oakland, CA: New Harbinger.

Greenberger, D., & Padesky, C. A. (2016). *Mind over mood: Change how you feel by changing the way you think* (2nd ed.). New York: Guilford Press.

Hofmann, S. G. (2020). *The anxiety skills workbook: Simple CBT and mindfulness strategies for overcoming anxiety, fear, and worry.* Oakland, CA: New Harbinger.

Kabat-Zinn, J. (2013). *Full catastrophe living: Using the wisdom of your body and mind to face stress, pain, and illness* (rev. ed.). New York: Bantam Books/Random House.

McKay, M., Davis, M., & Fanning, P. (2018). *Messages: The communications skills book* (4th ed.). Oakland, CA: New Harbinger.

Orsillo, S. M., & Roemer, L. (2016). *Worry less, live more: The mindful way through anxiety workbook.* New York: Guilford Press.

Anxiety Disorders in Children and Adolescents (for Parents)

Eisen, A. R., & Engler, L. B. (2006). *Helping your child with separation anxiety: A step-by-step guide for parents*. Oakland, CA: New Harbinger.

Foa, E. B., & Andrews, L. W. (2006). *If your adolescent has an anxiety disorder: An essential resource for parents*. New York: Oxford University Press.

Freeman, J. B., & Garcia, A. M. (2009). *Family-based treatment for young children with OCD (workbook)*. New York: Oxford University Press.

Josephs, S. A. (2017). *Helping your anxious teen: Positive parenting strategies to help your teen beat anxiety, stress, and worry*. Oakland, CA: New Harbinger.

Kearney, C. A. (2011). *Silence is not golden: Strategies for helping the shy child*. New York: Oxford University Press.

Kearney, C. A., & Albano, A. M. (2007). *When children refuse school: A cognitive behavioral therapy approach* (parent workbook). New York: Oxford University Press.

March, J. S., & Benton, C. M. (2007). *Talking back to OCD: The program that helps kids and teens say "no way"—and parents say "way to go."* New York: Guilford Press.

McHolm, A. E., Cunningham, C. E., & Vanier, M. K. (2005). *Helping your child with selective mutism: Practical steps to overcome a fear of speaking*. Oakland, CA: New Harbinger.

Rapee, R. M., Spence, S. H., Cobham, V., Wignall, A., & Lyneham, H. (2008). *Helping your anxious child: A step-by-step guide for parents* (2nd ed.). Oakland, CA: New Harbinger.

Anxiety Disorders in Children and Adolescents (for Children and Adolescents)

Alter, R., & Clarke, C. (2016). *The anxiety workbook for kids: Take charge of fears and worries using the gift of imagination*. Oakland, CA: New Harbinger.

Brozovich, R., & Chase, L. (2008). *Say goodbye to being shy: A workbook to help kids overcome shyness*. Oakland, CA: Instant Help Books.

Ehrenreich-May, J., Kennedy, S. M., Sherman, J. A., Bennett, S. M., & Barlow, D. H. (2018). *Unified protocols for transdiagnostic treatment of emotional disorders in adolescents: Workbook*. New York: Oxford University Press.

Khanna, M. S., & Ledley, D. R. (2018). *The worry workbook for kids: Helping children to overcome anxiety and the fear of uncertainty*. Oakland, CA: New Harbinger.

Piacentini, J., Langley, A., & Roblek, T. (2007). *It's only a false alarm* (workbook). New York: Oxford University Press.

Tompkins, M. A., & Martinez, K. (2010). *My anxious mind: A teen's guide to managing anxiety and panic*. Washington, DC: Magination Press.

Panic Disorder and Agoraphobia

Antony, M. M., & McCabe, R. E. (2004). *10 simple solutions to panic: How to overcome panic attacks, calm physical symptoms, and reclaim your life*. Oakland, CA: New Harbinger.

Barlow, D. H., & Craske, M. G. (2007). *Mastery of your anxiety and panic: Workbook* (4th ed.). New York: Oxford University Press.

Wilson, R. (2009). *Don't panic: Taking control of anxiety attacks* (3rd ed.). New York: HarperCollins.

Social Anxiety

Antony, M. M. (2004). *10 simple solutions to shyness: How to overcome shyness, social anxiety, and fear of public speaking.* Oakland, CA: New Harbinger. Available as a free PDF download at *http://martinantony.com/publications* (click on "Downloads").

Antony, M. M., & Swinson, R. P. (2017). *The shyness and social anxiety workbook: Proven, step-by-step techniques for overcoming your fear* (3rd ed.). Oakland, CA: New Harbinger.

Butler, G. (2016). *Overcoming social anxiety and shyness: A self-help guide using cognitive behavioral techniques* (2nd ed.). London, UK: Little, Brown.

Fleming, J. E., & Kocovski, N. L. (2013). *The mindfulness and acceptance workbook for social anxiety and shyness: Using acceptance and commitment therapy to free yourself from fear and reclaim your life.* Oakland, CA: New Harbinger.

Hope, D. A., Heimberg, R. G., & Turk, C. L. (2019). *Managing social anxiety: A cognitive behavioral therapy approach* (3rd ed.) (workbook). New York: Oxford University Press.

Monarth, H., & Kase, L. (2007). *The confident speaker: Beat your nerves and communicate at your best in any situation.* New York: McGraw-Hill.

Generalized Anxiety Disorder and Chronic Worry

Gyoerkoe, K. L., & Wiegartz, P. S. (2006). *10 simple solutions to worry: How to calm your mind, relax your body, and reclaim your life.* Oakland, CA: New Harbinger.

Meares, K., & Freeston, M. (2015). *Overcoming worry and generalized anxiety disorder: A self-help guide using cognitive behavioral techniques* (2nd ed.). London: Robinson Press.

Robichaud, M. R., & Buhr, K. (2018). *The worry workbook: CBT skills to overcome worry and anxiety by facing the fear of uncertainty.* Oakland, CA: New Harbinger.

Robichaud, M. R., & Dugas, M. J. (2015). *The generalized anxiety disorder workbook: A comprehensive CBT guide for coping with uncertainty, worry, and fear.* Oakland, CA: New Harbinger.

Specific Fears and Phobias

Antony, M. M., Craske, M. G., & Barlow, D. H. (2006). *Mastering your fears and phobias* (2nd ed.) (workbook). New York: Oxford University Press.

Antony, M. M., & McCabe, R. E. (2005). *Overcoming animal and insect phobias: How to conquer fear of dogs, snakes, rodents, bees, spiders, and more.* Oakland, CA: New Harbinger. Available as a free PDF download at *http://martinantony.com/publications* (click on "Downloads").

Antony, M. M., & Rowa, K. (2007). *Overcoming fear of heights: How to conquer acrophobia and live a life without limits.* Oakland, CA: New Harbinger. Available as a free PDF download at *http://martinantony.com/publications* (click on "Downloads").

Antony, M. M., & Watling, M. (2006). *Overcoming medical phobias: How to conquer fear of blood, needles, doctors, and dentists.* Oakland, CA: New Harbinger. Available as a free PDF download at *http://martinantony.com/publications* (click on "Downloads").

Brown, D. (2009). *Flying without fear: Effective strategies to get you where you want to go* (2nd ed.). Oakland, CA: New Harbinger.

Carbonell, D. (2017). *Fear of flying workbook: Overcome your anticipatory anxiety and develop skills for flying with confidence.* Berkeley, CA: Ulysses Press.

Triffitt, J. (2003). *Back in the driver's seat: Understanding, challenging, and managing fear of driving.* Tasmania, Australia: Author. Available at *www.backinthedriversseat.com.au.*

Obsessive–Compulsive Disorder

Abramowitz, J. S. (2018). *Getting over OCD: A 10-step workbook for taking back your life* (2nd ed.). New York: Guilford Press.

Baer, L. (2012). *Getting control: Overcoming your obsessions and compulsions* (3rd ed.). New York: Plume.

Challacombe, F., Oldfield, V. B., & Salkovskis, P. (2011). *Break free from OCD: Overcoming obsessive compulsive disorder with CBT.* London: Vermilion.

Grayson, J. (2014). *Freedom from obsessive–compulsive disorder: A personalized recovery program for living with uncertainty* (rev. ed.). New York: Berkley.

Hyman, B. M., & Pedrick, C. (2010). *The OCD workbook: Your guide to breaking free from obsessive–compulsive disorder* (3rd ed.). Oakland, CA: New Harbinger.

Purdon, C., & Clark, D. A. (2005). *Overcoming obsessive thoughts: How to gain control of your OCD.* Oakland, CA: New Harbinger.

Winston, S. M., & Seif, M. N. (2017). *Overcoming unwanted intrusive thoughts: A CBT-based guide to getting over frightening obsessive, or disturbing thoughts.* Oakland, CA: New Harbinger.

Yadin, E., Foa, E. B., & Lichner, T. K. (2012). *Treating your OCD with exposure and response (ritual) prevention for obsessive–compulsive disorder* (2nd ed.) (workbook). New York: Oxford University Press.

Hoarding

Steketee, G., & Frost, R. O. (2014). *Treatment for hoarding disorder* (2nd ed.) (workbook). New York: Oxford University Press.

Tolin, D., Frost, R. O., & Steketee, G. (2014). *Buried in treasures: Help for compulsive acquiring, saving, and hoarding* (2nd ed.). New York: Oxford University Press.

Tolin, D. F., Worden, B. L., Wooton, B. M., & Gilliam, C. (2017). *CBT for hoarding disorder: A group therapy program* (workbook). Hoboken, NJ: Wiley Blackwell.

Tompkins, M. A., & Hartl, T. L. (2009). *Digging out: Helping your loved one manage clutter, hoarding, and compulsive acquiring.* Oakland, CA: New Harbinger.

Health Anxiety, Hair Pulling, Skin Picking, and Body Dysmorphic Disorder

Asmundson, G. J. G., & Taylor, S. (2005). *It's not all in your head: How worrying about your health could be making you sick—and what you can do about it.* New York: Guilford Press.

Mansueto, C. S., Vavrichek, S. M., & Golomb, R. (2020). *Overcoming body-focused repetitive behaviors: A comprehensive behavioral treatment for hair pulling and skin picking.* Oakland, CA: New Harbinger.

Owens, K. M. B., & Antony, M. M. (2011). *Overcoming health anxiety: Letting go of your fear of illness.* Oakland, CA: New Harbinger.

Wilhelm, S. (2006). *Feeling good about the way you look: A program for overcoming body image problems.* New York: Guilford Press.

Trauma and Posttraumatic Stress Disorder

Back, S. E., Foa, E. B., et al. (2014). *Concurrent treatment for PTSD and substance use disorders with prolonged exposure (COPE)* (patient workbook). New York: Oxford University Press.

Hickling, E. J., & Blanchard, E. B. (2006). *Overcoming the trauma of your motor vehicle accident: A cognitive-behavioral treatment program* (workbook). New York: Oxford University Press.

Rothbaum, B. O., Foa, E. B., Hembree, E. A., & Rauch, S. A. M. (2019). *Reclaiming your life from a traumatic experience* (2nd ed.) (workbook). New York: Oxford University Press.

Tull, M. T., Gratz, K. L., & Chapman, A. L. (2016). *Cognitive-behavioral coping skills workbook for PTSD: Overcome fear and anxiety and reclaim your life.* Oakland, CA: New Harbinger.

Depression

Addis, M. E., & Martell, C. R. (2004). *Overcoming depression one step at a time: The new behavioral activation approach to getting your life back.* Oakland, CA: New Harbinger.

Paterson, R. J. (2016). *How to be miserable: 40 strategies you already use.* Oakland, CA: New Harbinger.

Strosahl, K. D., & Robinson, P. J. (2017). *The mindfulness and acceptance workbook for depression: Using acceptance and commitment therapy to move through depression and create a life worth living* (2nd ed.). Oakland, CA: New Harbinger.

Teasdale, J., Williams, M., & Segal, Z. (2014). *The mindful way workbook: An 8-week program to free yourself from depression and emotional distress.* New York: Guilford Press.

Williams, M., Teasdale, J., & Segal, Z. (2007). *The mindful way through depression.* New York: Guilford Press.

Wright, J. H., & McCray, L. W. (2012). *Breaking free from depression: Pathways to wellness.* New York: Guilford Press.

Perfectionism

Antony, M. M., & Swinson, R. P. (2009). *When perfect isn't good enough: Strategies for coping with perfectionism* (2nd ed.). Oakland, CA: New Harbinger.

Shafran, R., Egan, S., & Wade, T. (2018). *Overcoming perfectionism: A self-help guide using cognitive behavioural techniques* (2nd ed.). London: Robinson Press.

Index

about the authors

Peter J. Norton, PhD, is Professor of Psychology and Associate Head of School (Research) at the Cairnmillar Institute in Melbourne, Australia. A Fellow of the American Psychological Association, Dr. Norton is an internationally recognized researcher and developer of transdiagnostic cognitive-behavioral therapy for emotional disorders.

Martin M. Antony, PhD, is Professor of Psychology at Ryerson University in Toronto, Canada. An internationally known expert on anxiety and related topics, Dr. Antony is a past president of the Canadian Psychological Association and the Association for Behavioral and Cognitive Therapies, and is a Fellow of the Royal Society of Canada.

list of audio tracks

Track 1	Progressive Muscle Relaxation—Long Form	24:40
Track 2	Progressive Muscle Relaxation—Short Form	14:12
Track 3	Progressive Muscle Relaxation—Full Body	3:10